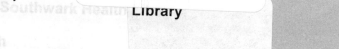
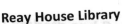
TACKLING TEENAGE PREGNANCY

SEX, CULTURE AND NEEDS

Ruth Chambers, Gill Wakley and
Steph Chambers

With contributions from
Anna Brown

Foreword by
Cathy Hamlyn
Head of the Teenage Pregnancy Unit
Department of Health

RADCLIFFE MEDICAL PRESS

Radcliffe Medical Press Ltd
18 Marcham Road, Abingdon, Oxon OX14 1AA

British Library Cataloguing in Publication Data

A catalogue record for this book is available from the British Library.

ISBN 1 85775 497 2

Typeset by Aarontype Ltd., Easton, Bristol
Printed and bound by TJ International Ltd, Padstow, Cornwall

► CONTENTS

► FOREWORD

Over the last couple of years, Britain has woken up to its high pregnancy rate and to the problems this causes individuals and wider society. A lively debate is now taking place about the best way to tackle teenage pregnancy and minimise the risks of social exclusion for teenage parents and their children. But we already know that among the different approaches to improving services there are a few basic principles:

- listen to young people themselves
- join up services and professionals
- don't repeat past mistakes but build on what has been shown to succeed.

This book builds on those principles and it uses young people's voices to clarify how they can be helped to make informed choices about their health and their futures.

It is a timely, valuable addition to the literature and the learning on this subject.

Cathy Hamlyn
Head of the Teenage Pregnancy Unit
Department of Health
October 2000

▶ PREFACE

The problem of unplanned teenage pregnancies requires a change in culture so that we adopt a more holistic approach to teenagers' sexual health and recognise everyone's contribution to tackling the problem.

There are opportunities for those employed at local level in the health service, the education sector, the voluntary sector and leisure/sports organisations to work together. They should try to find approaches that make more of an impact on teenagers' sexual behaviour by offering support, providing practical information and making services and education more appropriate to young people's needs.

Throughout the text we have referred to 'family planning clinics' as this is the term with which most readers are familiar. These might be better termed 'contraception and advice clinics' or 'sexual health clinics' in future.

This book will extend professionals' knowledge, skills and attitudes with regard to interacting with young people. It will help professionals to understand both young people's thinking and the confused and conflicting messages that face teenagers today. Anna's thoughtful comments which follow illustrate very well some of the origins of that confusion.

Ruth Chambers
Gill Wakley
October 2000

A teenager's viewpoint

Anna Brown

Contraception

I believe that, at 16-years-old, I know the basics of sex and the consequences that are possible and even probable. However, even armed with this information there are still problems I have to undergo and risks I take, so there is still the chance of getting pregnant or contracting sexually transmitted diseases (STDs).

Different types of contraception are open to a person of my age, but with each method there are problems that must be overcome.

Condoms

Condoms can be easily obtained by most teenagers from Boots or any other chemist, but they are expensive, and if you are in a position where you are frequently sexually active, then the price mounts up to be unaffordable. Because of this problem, many teenagers may feel that they can no longer practise safe sex, so increasing the chance of pregnancy. Many say that the solution to this is to obtain condoms from a local Family Planning Centre where condoms can be obtained free of charge, but many teenagers then ask the same question 'Where is my local Family Planning Centre?'. From my point of view this information has to be made much more widely available.

When people do not use condoms they may be under the impression that if the man withdraws before ejaculation occurs then they will not be open to the risks of pregnancy or STDs. Information about the risks of getting pregnant from pre-ejaculation should be more clear and understandable.

The pill

The pill is considered by many young people to be a solution to all problems and worries about pregnancy, but this is simply not true, and the risks and consequences of incorrect usage have to be understood. This information can be provided through leaflets, but these have to be available where young people can obtain them without embarrassment.

Many girls all over the country become sexually active before they reach 16 years of age, but many doctors are reluctant – and sometimes refuse – to provide the pill to young girls, and therefore deny them this form of contraception. This problem needs to be addressed, because if contraception is not universally available to girls under 16-years-old, teenage pregnancy rates may stay the same or continue to rise.

Another point about the pill is the fact that many teenage girls are embarrassed about or afraid of going to see their doctor. They fear that their GP will either tell their parents about their requests, reprimand them or tell them they are stupid to be sexually active. Moreover, many young girls believe it is illegal to go on the pill before they are 16-years-old, and this is another reason that they wait – a wait which may be too long for some people. Girls need to be reassured about their right to privacy and assured that their GP will not embarrass them.

The morning-after pill

The morning-after pill could be a lifeline for many young girls, but it is sometimes impossible for them to go to their GP to obtain due to their being physically unable to get there. Once again there is the embarrassment of going to see their GP before they are 16-years-old and the worry of what they have to do to obtain the morning-after pill, which should be available over the counter at chemist shops, as the checks the doctors make can also be done by a pharmacist. This would help the fight against teenage pregnancy as, if a girl knows she has had unprotected sex and is at risk, then getting the morning-after pill may be essential for her, but if she has no way of getting to her GP she may well become pregnant. The morning-after pill is vital as a means of decreasing the number of teenage pregnancies, and it is truly a 'last chance' for many girls, but the problems of obtaining it within such a limited time span are such that it should be made more widely available and obtainable over the counter. One problem with the morning-after pill is that some people may use it as a substitute for regular contraception, but this can be overcome with education and the explanation that it is by no means a foolproof method, and that alternative contraception must therefore be planned and used.

Other forms of contraception

Other forms of contraception, such as the female condom or the diaphragm, are not particularly accessible to young people for many of the same reasons as the pill. Going to see your GP before you are 16-years-old can be embarrassing, and the GP may refuse to help you. Moreover, the condom is the form of contraception that most young couples use, if they are using any contraception at all. It should be made easier for young people to obtain information on this subject, describing each of the different available methods of contraceptions including where to get them and the side-effects that may occur.

Information about other forms of contraception should be made clearer to younger members of the public by means of leaflets and the Internet, as these provide a non-embarrassing way to obtain information.

Information

The only embarrassing thing about finding a leaflet and reading it is the actual act of obtaining it. Therefore leaflets should be sent to schools to be given out during personal and social education (PSE) and sexual education classes. Another way of providing information is through discussions between people who have plenty of information on the subject of contraception and a group of young teenagers. This would demonstrate to the informed person the delusions of the young about contraception, and would also inform the young in a very open and easy manner about ways to avoid risk. A well-designed leaflet is an effective way to provide accessible, factual information. Wider access to the Internet could also provide a very effective way of distributing information in the near future.

'Why am I listening to this, anyway? It will never happen to me!'

This is a delusion of many young people, and it is essential that it is overcome. One way to do this is to ask young people who either have babies or have been pregnant to come and talk to other teenagers of a similar age about their experiences. If teenagers hear about the experiences of other young people who had the same opinion – that it would never happen to them – then they may well sit up and take notice. Another way of showing how difficult it is to care for a baby when you are young and financially unstable involves taking a 'computerised baby' home for the night. This demonstrates how difficult it really is to be the parent of a young child, especially if the father and mother are no longer together. The doll may cry at any time of the night or day, and so highlights the fact that sleep is limited, and it also demonstrates the restriction of freedom that is caused by having a baby.

Peer pressure

Peer pressure has been around for a long time, and is a major reason why people have sex at such a young age and therefore put themselves at risk very early on in their lives. There is a practically non-existent chance of eradicating peer pressure, but it has to combated in some way. The best way to do this is by increasing awareness through education and personal experience, as talked about in previous sections. By making the young very aware of the risks and all of the possible outcomes of having sex early on in their lives, you are unlikely to stop them having sex, but you should increase the use of contraception and therefore reduce the risks. Many people have sex before they are ready because of pressure from friends or their partner, but a reduction in the number of teenage pregnancies should be possible, both by making them aware of the risks and also by providing free contraception.

Roman Catholic schools and their problems

Because Roman Catholic schools uphold the beliefs and morals of the Roman Catholic faith, few of them provide sex education for the simple reason that it goes against their beliefs, although ignoring the subject is very dangerous in today's world. The young people who attend these schools are highly likely to have sex as teenagers before they get married, but they will do so at a greater risk to themselves due to lack of informative education about the subject.

I myself go to a Roman Catholic school where they talk about sex in biology lessons but do not cover contraception in any detail at all. This is a very bad situation, because had my parents not been open about discussing sex and educated me as they saw fit, then I would have very little idea how to remain safe and reduce the risks. Many of the girls at school joke about sex, but they do not know how to remain safe. It is an amusing thing to them, but because they are not particularly aware of the risks they are in danger. Something has to be done to change this situation, maybe by making it compulsory to provide sex education and to emphasise safety in all schools. Many girls and boys who attend Roman Catholic schools go into sexual relationships blind, and this could result in many unwanted pregnancies and the passing on of STDs. However, with education of the schools, the teachers and most importantly the students, this path to teenage pregnancy could be reduced by passing on the simplest information.

► ABOUT THE AUTHORS

Ruth Chambers has been a GP for 21 years. Her previous experience has encompassed a wide range of research and educational activities, including stress and the health of doctors, the quality of healthcare and many other topics.

She is currently the Professor of Primary Care Development at the School of Health at Staffordshire University. As Chair of Staffordshire Medical Audit Advisory Group Ruth led a district-wide audit of contraceptive services for teenagers in the 1990s, involving general practices, family planning clinics and maternity/termination services in the acute sector. Many gaps in services were identified, but few of them were rectified. Hopefully a culture of clinical governance will increase local determination to realign resources to respond to teenagers' needs.

Gill Wakley started in general practice in 1966, but transferred to community medicine shortly afterwards and then into public health. A desire for increased contact with patients caused her to move back into general practice, together with community gynaecology, in 1978. She has been combining the two areas of medicine in varying ratios ever since.

Throughout her career Gill has been heavily involved in learning and teaching. She was in a training general practice, became an instructing doctor and a regional assessor in family planning, and was until recently a Senior Clinical Lecturer with the Primary Care Department at Keele University. Like Ruth, she has run all types of educational initiatives and activities, ranging from individual mentoring and instruction to small group work, plenary lectures, distance learning programmes, workshops, and courses for a wide range of health professionals and lay people.

Steph Chambers is a teenager aged 14 years who has opinions on most subjects. She brings the fresh perspective of a teenager to the problems that beset teenage sexuality and lead to unplanned pregnancies and sexually transmitted diseases. Her ideas and critique should add new insight to help us to understand how we should modify our approaches to young people so as to help them to make informed choices.

Anna Brown is 16-years-old and attends a girls' school run by the Roman Catholic church. Her frustration with the way in which the school ignores issues surrounding teenage sexuality is apparent in the preface to this book. Like Steph, Anna is a member of a young people's group that advises about the direction of an educational project led by Ruth Chambers, with the aim of finding new ways to reduce the number of unplanned teenage pregnancies.

▶ ACKNOWLEDGEMENTS

Our enthusiasm for writing this book has arisen from our wish to inform and empower the very many teenagers whom we have met in the course of our work who have found themselves having to cope with unplanned pregnancies. Much of the momentum for writing the book was fuelled by the Health Action Zone Innovations Project in North Staffordshire, which has been funded by the Department of Health and is led by Ruth Chambers. We have drawn ideas from the 12 young people who constitute an advisory group to the project, and from the doctors, nurses, social workers, youth workers and others who are involved in different ways.

We are grateful to Alison Hadley, specialist policy and implementation manager at the Teenage Pregnancy Unit, for her suggestions and proofreading.

▶ CHAPTER 1

Introduction

Reducing teenage conception rates and preventing unwanted pregnancies across all age groups is a key national priority. Teenage conception rates in the UK continue to be the highest in Western Europe, despite the many local programmes that were set up to meet the original *Health of the Nation* target of 1990, namely to halve conception rates in those under 16 years of age by the year 2000.[1]

However, whilst the rate of unplanned teenage pregnancies has remained at a steady value, the mean age of mothers at birth has been steadily increasing over the last 30 years, so that it is now 29 years in England, Scotland and Northern Ireland and 28 years in Wales.[2]

Why do young people have unprotected sex?

Most sexually active teenagers do not become pregnant, and more than two-thirds of young people aged under 16 years of age do not have sex. Therefore we should find ways to help to prevent pregnancy in the cohort that is most likely to be at risk of having unprotected sexual intercourse. It is thought that young people do not use contraception because they have problems finding and accessing traditional sexual health services, they are anxious about confidentiality and legality, and they are ignorant about using contraception.[3,4]

One survey showed that 45% of teenage girls who were sexually experienced had had unprotected sex, a fifth had not used contraceptives at first intercourse, and one-third of the girls had used emergency contraception.[5]

In an American survey[6] of 515 teenagers aged 12 to 17 years, more than half of the respondents stated that the main reason why young people do not use birth control was due to drinking alcohol or using drugs (boys and girls gave similar answers). Half of the teenagers who were questioned thought another common reason for young people having unprotected sex was pressure from partners who did not want to use contraception. Young adolescents aged 12 to 14 years were as likely to say this as the older teenagers.

A comprehensive report by the Social Exclusion Unit attributes the high rates of teenage conception in the UK to young people's low expectations, ignorance about contraception and what is involved in forming relationships and parenting, and mixed messages ('it sometimes seems as if sex is compulsory but contraception is illegal').[3]

The scale of the problem

In England, nearly 90 000 conceptions occur in teenagers per year, 7700 to girls aged under 16 years and 2200 to girls aged 14 years or younger. About 60% (56 000) of those conceptions result in live births. The conception rate for women aged 15 to 19 years was 64.9 per 1000 women in 1996.[2] Just over 15 000 of those under 18 years old had a termination. Termination is the option chosen by about half of those under 16 years old and more than one-third of 16- and 17-year-olds.[3]

The latest figures (for the year 2000) from the Office of National Statistics[2] showed that just over 90% of conceptions within marriage resulted in maternity, compared to two-thirds of conceptions outside marriage. The proportion of conceptions outside marriage was 51% in 1998, and 90% of teenage mothers have their babies outside marriage. Relationships that start during teenage years have at least a 50% chance of breaking down, leaving a high proportion of lone parents.

The area of most concern is the rate of conceptions among those under 16-years-old, in whom maternal and fetal risks are highest. The death rate for babies of teenage mothers is 60% higher than that for babies of older mothers.

Comparisons with Europe

Teenage birth rates in the UK are twice as high as those in Germany, three times as high as those in France and six times higher than those in The Netherlands.

The European Commission reports on the state of health of young people (aged 15 to 24 years) in the European Union, and on the extent of risk-taking behaviour.[7] They monitor the status of *reproductive health* among young people by levels of unintended pregnancies and *sexually transmitted diseases* (STDs). Chlamydia is by far the most common of the sexually transmitted diseases, and is carried by 5–7% of young people in Europe. Between 1992 and 1997 the annual number of new cases of AIDS in the 15–24 years age group decreased from about 1050 cases to about 460 cases. The frequency of smoking, alcohol consumption and substance abuse by children and young people is increasing: 50–80% of children aged 15 years have tried smoking, and about 20% of all 15-year-olds were reported to be daily cigarette smokers in 1988. Drinking to inebriation has become increasingly common among young people, and the rate of use of cannabis ranged from 4% to 41% across the European Union among those aged 15–16 years in the mid-1990s.

We need to consider ways to reduce the incidence of unplanned pregnancy against the general background of risk-seeking behaviour being a normal part of adolescence, and by understanding the *social, economic and cultural determinants of health* which lead to increasing inequalities in young people's health.

Throughout the 1990s, *teenage fertility rates* have been generally decreasing across the European Union.[7] The largest decreases in teenage fertility rates have been reported from Greece (−76%), Spain (−59%) and Finland (−57%), whereas only in the UK, Denmark, The Netherlands and Ireland are the rates of the mid-1990s at about the same level as those of the mid-1980s (*see* Table 1.1).

In 1995, the teenage fertility rate was lowest in The Netherlands (4 live births per 1000 women) and highest in the UK (23 per 1000) and Portugal (17 per 1000), with a

Table 1.1: Comparison of live birth rates in girls aged 15 to 19 years, between 1986 and 1996[7]

	Live birth rates (per 1000 females)	
Country	1986	1996
Iceland	39.3	16.3
Greece	25.9	9.6
UK	23.9	22.9
Portugal	24.2	16.6
Austria	17.8	11.5
France	10.7	6.8
Norway	13.4	9.9
Ireland	12.4	12.7*
Sweden	7.9	5.5
Finland	9.5	6.9
Spain	13.1	6.1
Denmark	6.7	5.7
Germany	13.0	9.6
Luxembourg	6.7	7.0
The Netherlands	5.1	4.1

* provisional

Table 1.2: Termination of pregnancy rates in 1996, according to country (age < 20 years)[7]

Country	Termination rates per 1000 women
England and Wales	21.7
Sweden	17.8
Denmark	15.9
Finland	9.6
Belgium	5.9
Spain	4.9
Greece	1.3

European Union average of 10 live births per 1000 women. The highest *teenage* abortion rates per 1000 women were reported from England and Wales (22 per 1000), Sweden (18 per 1000) and Denmark (16 per 1000), and the lowest rates were reported from Spain (5 per 1000) and Belgium (6 per 1000) (*see* Table 1.2).

Social, cultural and economic determinants of health create inequalities and unequal opportunities for young people

Pregnant teenagers are more likely than mothers aged 20 to 35 years to have low income and poor education, be unmarried, be cigarette smokers and have poor nutrition. The Acheson Report[4] on health inequalities recognised that teenage mothers and their children are at higher risk of experiencing adverse health, educational, social and economic outcomes compared to older mothers and their children. The report called for policies which promote sexual health in young people and access to appropriate contraceptive services, so reducing the number of unwanted teenage pregnancies. The government's Social Exclusion Unit has responded by emphasising the need for 'joined up action' at local and national levels.[3]

Teenage pregnancy has been clearly highlighted as a key inequality issue.[8] However, a recent nationwide survey found that only 25% of health improvement programmes had developed a local focus on sexual health and teenage pregnancy rates through multi-agency working.[9]

There are many teenage boys like Ed, described below, living in deprived communities in the UK.

> There are boys who know no childhood; often they come from broken families, and end up barely literate, uncontrolled and uncontrollable ... Ed is 15 going on 20 ... He has played truant since primary school and is (probably) about to be a father ... 'I didn't mean to sleep with her (he said to a reporter), I got drunk' ... He is shamelessly promiscuous and has regular AIDS test 'to be on the safe side' ... Asked why his life was such a mess, Ed said 'It all boils down to trying to be hard. You've got to prove yourself to everybody, haven't you?'[10]

Risk factors for teenage pregnancy[3]

Teenage pregnancy is both a cause and an effect of inequalities in health.[3,4] Teenage mothers tend to have poor antenatal care, low birthweight infants and higher infant mortality rates. Teenage parents tend to miss out on education and to have substantially lower incomes. They are also more likely to suffer from postnatal depression and relationship breakdown. Risk factors for teenage pregnancy include having a teenage mother, having divorced parents, deprivation, being a child living in care, educational problems, sexual abuse, ethnicity, mental health problems and crime. A brief description of some of these factors follows.

- *Poverty*: the risk of becoming a teenage mother is almost ten times higher for a girl whose family is in social class V (unskilled, manual) than for one whose family is in social class I (professional).[3]

- *Children in care or leaving care*: one study found that women who had been in care or fostered were more than twice as likely to become teenage mothers as those who had been brought up by both natural parents. Another study found that nearly 50% of girls leaving care became mothers within 18 to 24 months.[3]
- *Children of teenage mothers*: the daughter of a teenage mother is 1.5 times more likely to become a teenage mother herself than is the daughter of an older mother.[3]
- *Low educational achievement*: a significant proportion of teenage mothers leave school with no qualifications (40% in one study). Girls who truant or who are excluded from school are at high risk.[3]
- *Not being in education, training or work after 16 years of age*.[3]
- *Sexual abuse*: it may be that young people lack the confidence to resist sexual pressure, even years after the abuse took place.[3]
- *Mental health problems*: there may be a link between mental health problems and increased likelihood of teenage pregnancy.[3]
- *Crime*: one study found that teenagers who had been in trouble with the police were twice as likely to become teenage parents as those who had had no contact with the police.[3]

The effect of risk factors for teenage pregnancy may be cumulative. Some ethnic groups are over-represented in the various at-risk categories. For instance, disproportionately more African-Caribbean, Pakistani and Bangladeshi people are in low-income groups compared to white people.

Cost-effectiveness of preventing unwanted pregnancies

Estimates of cost savings of £377 to £466 per unwanted pregnancy avoided (for clinic and general practice provision,

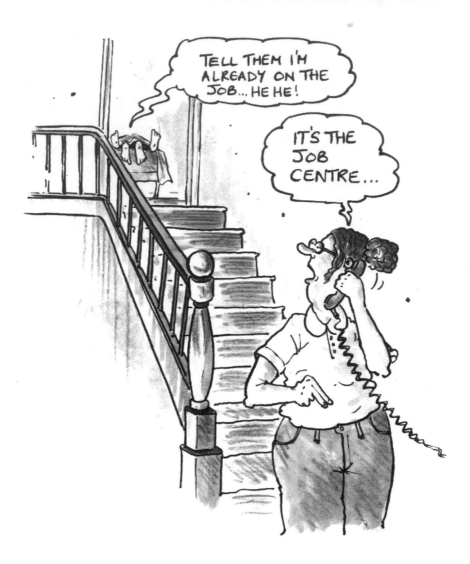

respectively) indicate that the provision of contraceptive services to teenagers is highly cost-effective.[4] Moreover, longer term health gains obtained by avoiding the poor health and sequelae of teenage mothers and their babies as the family grows up mean that these cost savings are in reality much greater. Women who do not have babies while they are teenagers have more opportunities to gain qualifications and train for a career, making claims for benefit at a later date less likely – another financial saving.

A selection of young people's views about sex, contraception and school education

The following report has been written by Steph Chambers, and reflects the views of many of her contemporaries

'I just reckon that young people at the age of 16 or under should use protection because they are too young to have babies and they might not be able to afford to look after their baby/babies properly.'

(18-year-old girl attending university)

'I think teenagers won't be discouraged by adults or the law telling them that having sex is wrong. They need to be made aware of all the facts and possibilities of teenage pregnancy and need the education of it all when they are much younger, at about the age of seven or eight years old. When they are that age, much more definite information should be given. It should be much more explicit in terms of contraception. The different options that there are if they do get pregnant should also be a main topic.'

(14-year-old girl attending independent school)

'I think that I would've preferred single-sex lessons at school, especially as boys don't have any other place to go for information. Girls have clinics and that, but nothing is set up for lads. But if there was, I think that almost all lads would be too embarrassed to use them anyway.'

(16-year-old boy attending comprehensive school)

'It might be easier if the receptionists at my local GPs weren't so inquisitive. There aren't many women GPs available, and I'd feel more comfortable if the doctor was young.'

(15-year-old girl attending comprehensive school)

'I would feel uncomfortable going to the doctors' to ask for the emergency pill because if I was to go back there with

continued

my mum if I wasn't very well, then she would be able to see my medical notes if the computer screen was pointing towards us.'

(15-year-old girl attending comprehensive school)

'I think the main reason why young girls have sex is because of the pressure exerted by boys. If their friends are doing it, they don't have the confidence to say no.'

(17-year-old girl attending college)

'I think that teenage pregnancy is put down mainly to lads pressurising girls, but lads actually feel pressured into having sex as well. We also find it hard to talk about condoms and contraception to girls, but if we don't have sex then we can't talk about it when all our mates do.'

(16-year-old boy attending comprehensive school)

'I would find it difficult to talk to a GP because my dad is a part of the medical profession.'

(15-year-old girl attending comprehensive school)

'Under-age sex is not acknowledged at my school because it is a Catholic school. The school won't talk about it openly because the nuns think sex is wrong and cannot be contemplated.'

(15-year-old girl attending Catholic school)

'I don't think that there is a solution to teenage pregnancy, and no matter how hard professionals and people doing projects try, there will still be a larger proportion of girls who will not change. I'm not saying that all efforts will not have some kind of effect or anything, but under-age sex is some unwritten rule in the teenage mind. It goes down to teenagers sleeping with other teenagers because they feel that if they don't then they are somehow different to all their other mates and feel inferior. They cannot talk to their mates that have had sex, and they feel excluded.

continued

I think that if there was more sex education in my school or different projects set up in lessons such as English or Biology, then many girls in my class and year would have a much better in-depth understanding of under-age sex and the consequences.

Teachers have to realise what goes on out of school that involves teenage relationships. Teachers need to put young teenagers off under-age sex and also tell them where to find the relevant information if they were to contract an STD or even become pregnant. I think that teachers, especially in my school, have to understand that just because we pay to go there does not mean that we all sit at home doing our homework and behave out of school. After all, we're teenagers and have to enjoy life while we still can.

I don't think that girls that I'm friends with and others, certainly our age, want to sleep with boys. Some of my close friends have told me that it was a relief when they had done it and they didn't think it was such a big deal and why everyone was always on about it. One girl wished that she had waited until she was older and done it in her own time with the right person, so that she didn't feel so pressurised into it.'

(14-year-old girl attending independent school)

References

1   Department of Health (1993) *Health of the Nation: HIV/AIDS and Sexual Health*. The Stationery Office, London.

2   Office for National Statistics (2000) *Population Trends* 99. Government Statistical Service, The Stationery Office, London.

3   Department of Health (1999) *Teenage Pregnancy*. Social Exclusion Unit, Department of Health, London.

4 Acheson D (chair) (1998) *Independent Inquiry into Inequalities in Health Report*. The Stationery Office, London.

5 Chambers R and Milsom G (1995) *Audit of Contraceptive Services in Mid and North Staffordshire in Secondary Care, Primary Care and the Community*. Keele University, Keele.

6 National Campaign to Prevent Teen Pregnancy (2000) *Risky Business: a 2000 Poll*. National Campaign to Prevent Teen Pregnancy, Washington, DC.

7 European Commission (2000) *Report on the State of Young People's Health in the European Union: a Commission Services Working Paper*. European Commission, Brussels.

8 Department of Health (1999) *Saving Lives*. The Stationery Office, London.

9 Underdown A and Sexty C (2000) Getting the hump with HImPs. *Health Service J*. **27 Jan**: 22–24.

10 Chesshyre R (2000) So hard it hurts. *Telegraph Magazine* **27 May**: 36–43.

CHAPTER 2

Effective interventions and practical initiatives to reduce teenage pregnancy rates

Specific interventions will be most effective if they are designed to:

- take account of the local context and circumstances
- target those who are at most risk or who will benefit most
- be given at the most appropriate time, when they are likely to make most impact on the young person
- be relevant and acceptable to young people and the local community, whether they involve promotion of sexual health or contraception services
- be individualised for those with special needs (e.g. the gay and lesbian communities).[1]

There are two main approaches to reducing unintended teenage pregnancy rates – first, educational interventions, and second, the provision and delivery of contraceptive or sexual/relationship counselling services. A review of the evidence[2] of what works found that:

- school-based sex education can be effective, especially when linked to accessible contraceptive services
- contraceptive services should be based on an assessment of local needs, and be accessible and confidential

- the health and development of teenage mothers and their children benefit from programmes which promote access to antenatal care, targeted support by health visitors and social workers, and educational opportunities aimed at breaking the cycle of the daughters of teenage mothers being more likely to become teenage mothers themselves.

The following case history illustrates the multi-sectoral approach that is needed to address unplanned pregnancy.

The writer is a young person currently having unprotected sex herself

'*Availability of condoms*
Why can't boys get them from the GPs? Do boys attend family planning clinics? They should be encouraged to attend clinics and GPs themselves.

Sex education in schools
I attended XX High School and the sex education was dead basic. We had sessions once a week with the school nurse. Girls and boys had different sessions. I would have preferred it to be a joint session because I always sat with the lads, I get on with them better. It should be made more exciting than just advice about how to put a condom on. I don't like using condoms because I worry about them coming off, and I don't enjoy sex as much with them on; I don't like the smell and feel of them. I don't think about infections and things like AIDS and I have a partner who I've been with for a year now. I don't have sex with strangers so I don't worry. I didn't like school at all and I didn't listen to what the teachers had to say, so I don't really think school is the best place for sex education.

Contraception advice
I have been to a family planning clinic once and I don't intend to go again. I thought I was pregnant but they

continued

wouldn't do a test and just gave me condoms. I gave them away. I then went to my doctor for a test. The nurse was good. I think my GP listened to me properly and I felt like he cared about it. I was not embarrassed to talk to the doctor. I would feel more embarrassed going to the family planning clinic because everybody knows what you're there for. The waiting-room at YY clinic is the same one that is used for the baby clinic, and they have to walk right down the corridor and then I had to wait for the receptionist to give me the condoms (which I didn't even want!).

I don't use any contraception at the moment and I'm still not pregnant. I don't worry about it. If I was pregnant I wouldn't have a termination.'

(N, aged 18 years and unemployed)

Researchers have attempted to explain the very wide variation between the annual rates of teenage conception in different countries. They concluded that this variation was mainly due to how effectively teenagers use contraception, rather than to the extent of sexual activity. Three main factors seemed to be associated with how effectively contraception was used:

- the degree of openness about sexuality and the extent to which teenage sexuality was accepted by the adult community
- the availability of good-quality information and education about sexual matters
- the provision of high-quality, user-friendly clinical services for young people.[3]

The Mersey strategy for reducing the number of unplanned pregnancies strengthened the sexual health services and refocused on special groups of women such as young women, women with learning disabilities, those

continued

from ethnic minorities and women registered with a general practice without a woman doctor. Six general practices in each locality were recognised as having a special interest in providing contraception for young people. Family planning nurses were redeployed to these general practices from family planning clinics. Collaboration between the practices and local schools, youth and community services and the NHS in general led to a successful reduction in teenage conception rates.[3]

Sex and relationships education in schools

It is generally accepted that sex and relationships education for young people needs to be more positive and augmented by more open attitudes between parents, teachers and young people. A school policy on sex and relationships education should ensure the inclusion in the school curriculum of a well-informed approach to preventing teenage pregnancy. There is no evidence that provision of sex education at school hastens the onset of sexual experience.[2]

A video has been produced using teenage actors from a local high school in response to an audit of post-coital contraception that revealed shortcomings in young people's knowledge about prevention of pregnancy and access to contraceptive services. The video was developed for use as part of the personal and social education (PSE) schools programme alongside an updated and standardised teaching pack. The results of an evaluation showed that the video helped to prompt active discussion of topics which are usually difficult to approach, and that it informed the teenage audience.[4]

In one study, teenage respondents complained that sex education at school was 'too little, too late'. They thought that school-based sex education focused on the mechanics of sex and contraception, rather than on relationships and social skills. The teenagers felt that they already knew the information taught to them as school sex education. All of them would have liked teenage mothers to visit school classes to describe the reality of life with a baby.[5]

The A Pause project promotes sex and relationships education in schools

The *A Pause* (Added Power And Understanding in Sex Education) project was established in 1990 as a collaboration between teachers, health professionals and young people. Teachers deliver interactive sessions at various stages to 11- to 15-year-olds as part of the curriculum. Peer educators aged 16 to 19 years reinforce positive messages about sex and relationships. Evaluation of the project has demonstrated that pupils have gained knowledge and skills from it, as well as adopting more tolerant attitudes.[6]

A review of existing research came up with the following professional priorities for sex and relationships education in schools:

- such education should be initiated before young people are sexually active
- school policies and practices should be regularly refined in response to advice from health professionals and feedback from young people themselves
- educational programmes should constructively challenge female and male stereotypes
- teachers should have the information, skills, confidence, resources and support that they need to talk about sex with young people

- sex education should include opportunities to learn and practise communication, assertiveness and negotiation skills
- school policy and practice with regard to confidentiality must be clear
- sex and relationships education should include accurate information about where and when local contraception and sexual health services for young people are available, and should explain that contraceptive services are confidential and free.[6]

Sex education in schools – what young people think and need

The following commentary has been written by Steph Chambers, and reports the views of her contemporaries

There is great discussion about how much sex education children are receiving at school nowadays. The answer is plainly not enough. Young people from different schools have clearly stated that they have received few sex education lessons, if any.

The schools aren't teaching today's society what they need to know before they are sexually active. What young people are getting taught is information about sex that is usually already known to them.

Sex education starts at around Year 7 while pupils are aged between 11 and 12 years. At this stage schools only teach their students the absolute basics about how babies are produced and born. Even though this is judged to be important by young people I know, they think that this should be taught when pupils are much younger, as it common for students to become sexually active in Year 7.

We prefer classes of boys and girls to be separate. A teacher of the opposite sex teaching the children causes most embarrassment. We prefer to have a young member of staff involved as well.

continued

Pupils feel that teachers are embarrassed to teach some of the topics involved in sex education, and this produces a tense atmosphere during the lesson. This makes pupils feel uneasy, nervous and uncomfortable, and they do not feel that they can ask questions.

The teachers need to come to grips with today's slang words that are used in relation to sex, and often they do not understand what pupils want to know. This occurs in independent and religious schools in particular.

Much stronger views should be adopted to get the necessary facts across to children while they are still young. Sex education should stress the reality of under-age sex leading to teenage pregnancy, and should describe different methods of prevention of pregnancy. Schools should consider providing condoms for all pupils who want them, although this could also be seen as promoting under-age sex, by making it easier to obtain contraception.

The different contraceptives are not explained fully, and neither is information given about how to use family planning clinics or local GPs.

However, this cannot all be blamed on the school system. Pupils simply do not feel comfortable discussing sex-related matters with members of staff, and there is not a full guarantee that what they say will be kept completely confidential. Most teenagers I know think that teachers gossip in the staff-room. Embarrassment in such situations is only natural, and will prevent most pupils from asking the necessary questions. They also think that confiding about their sexual concerns might influence the way in which that teacher behaves towards them in a different lesson.

It is not an easy thing to admit that you do not understand an aspect of sex, especially in front of classmates, and all teenagers make out that they know all the facts about sex even if they do not.

continued

However, some schools have recognised the need for new methods. One such school has set up a drop-in clinic. It operates during Monday lunchtimes and is run by the school nurse. You do not have to give your name, and the nurse therefore cannot tell your teacher, and it has a guarantee of being completely confidential. It has already proved to be reasonably successful. Pupils do not go just for sex-related questions, but also for family problems, etc. Therefore other pupils would not know why they are going.

At that same school they have done projects on child development, one of which was a project concerning teenage myths. The schoolchildren researched and interviewed people and explained in full why the myths were untrue. They then did a presentation to the class.

Some schools are dedicating a topic in science to sex education, with an assessment test at the end. It was said that 'it was the first topic for which almost everybody got 100%'.

It is obvious that the original system of sex education in schools is not having enough influence on today's pupils, and teenagers are simply not learning the information that they need to know. The government needs to think of new schemes and work with young people to find a combination that will work, and which teenagers will find interesting and less embarrassing to use.

School-based education programmes should be linked to skills development such as enabling the postponement of sexual activity and contraceptive services, with health professionals visiting the school and contributing to the educational programme.

Outsiders coming into schools

The following commentary by Steph Chambers reports her peers' views

Teenagers like the idea of teenager mothers and professionals experienced in teenage pregnancy coming to schools to talk. It is a simple but effective way to point out the risks of under-age sex, and to provide accurate detailed information.

Professionals such as GPs and staff from family planning centres can describe different scenarios that they have encountered and that way pupils do not have to ask questions but can just listen to the options that they would have if they found themselves in a similar situation.

This is good because it saves the embarrassment of having to ask questions, and pupils are more likely to listen to the information given, if it comes from someone strange to the school, whom they are never likely to meet again. Without realising it, they will receive a lot of information that they will remember, and if it came to it then they would know where to go for help in that situation.

Teenage mothers visiting the school can share their experiences and describe how they have coped. They can outline how much they have had to give up and what pupils would have to give up if they were in that situation, too. They can share their regrets and support for those in the same situation, and emphasise to pupils that this is not an advisable path to go down.

The young people's view is that it is a better idea for teenage mothers to go into schools rather than health professionals, as the experiences of young mothers would be shocking and unusual. It would not be like other sex education lessons, and would be unlikely to be forgotten. Moreover, hearing the teenage mother's story and seeing

continued

living proof of their situation would be completely different to being told mere statistics by a teacher.

A previous project that has been published reported that 'All the teenage mothers interviewed said that they would discourage other teenagers from becoming pregnant (some were even prepared to get involved in school lessons to promote this)'. What we want to know is why this theory has not been put into practice.

Partnership working

Systematic reviews of the effectiveness of sexual health interventions aimed at young people recognise the social, educational, political and health dimensions that contribute to the causes of unwanted or unintended pregnancy and at which interventions are addressed.[2,7,8] Therefore, in order to be effective, interventions require multifaceted approaches and partnership working between the various organisations with a role in or responsibility for young people's health and well-being.

Effective local partnership working should include the teenagers themselves (both boys and girls), their parents, schoolteachers and nurses, health promotion facilitators, health professionals working in primary care and family planning services settings, social workers, community workers who work with underprivileged children and their families, the media and press, and those who plan and commission contraceptive services. There are organisational partnerships too, such as that between the health service and Social Services through the Sure Start Plus initiative. This will provide pregnant teenagers with impartial advice, and will help them to work through the options of keeping their babies, adoption or abortion, as well as providing wide-based support for teenage parents to help them to overcome disadvantage and poverty.

> Hodgehill Primary Care Group is working with a multi-agency group, consisting of representatives from the health improvement programme, the single regeneration bid project, the Education Action Zone and others, to tackle high teenage pregnancy rates in the locality by focusing on increasing young people's skills through peer education.

The success of the Dutch in achieving low teenage pregnancy rates, which are about one-sixth of the UK rates, demonstrates the potential effectiveness of partnership working, where parental influence, the importance of assertiveness training for children in primary schools, and the link to healthcare are all thought to contribute to the low teenage pregnancy rates and the average age of first intercourse being delayed to 17 years.

A total of 150 teenage pregnancy co-ordinators have been appointed in each local authority area in England in 2000.[9] The co-ordinators will lead the drive to implement the Social Exclusion Unit's report.[6] Most of the local co-ordinators are employed by health authorities to work with local authorities and all other organisations with a role in or responsibility for reducing teenage pregnancy, to develop a local strategy and action plan to meet national goals. These goals are to halve conception rates among young people under 18 years of age by 2010 and to get more teenage parents into education, training and employment. Their local strategies are expected to involve partners in reshaping contraceptive services to meet young people's needs, to advertise clinics' confidentiality policies and to support schools in delivering more effective education about sex and relationships.

> In Cornwall, the youth service, the health promotion service and the Barbican theatre in Plymouth are combining forces to increase young people's access to primary
>
> *continued*

care sexual health services. The project evolved from a theatre-in-education project working with primary healthcare teams. Other organisations have now been drawn into working on the initiative, including the local NHS (health authority, primary care groups and trusts), local education authority (including the out-of-school education service and Cornwall Association of Secondary Heads), Social Services, the child protection team, the county and district councils, housing, the NSPCC, Red Cross, youth agencies and many others. There have been many discussions and ongoing consultations with young people to ensure that the initiative is informed and led by them to create excellent health services for young people that promote health from a holistic point of view. A model of a young person-centred public health practitioner role is being developed and piloted in primary care.[10]

One evolving local strategy in Leicester City is typical of others. Teenage conception rates in the city are high, and the overall figure conceals a considerable range, with most conceptions occurring in wards in the west of the City with relatively high social deprivation indices. The key stakeholders in the Leicester City plan constitute a multi-agency teenage pregnancy group that includes representatives from health service strategic programmes and healthcare services with other non-health organisations or local improvement initiatives. The various partners are listed in the box below.

Strategies and partners in the Leicester City programme to reduce the teenage pregnancy rate

- Health improvement programme
- Children's strategy

continued

- Public health
- Health promotion
- Family planning services
- Genito-urinary medicine clinics
- Obstetric and gynaecology directorate
- Host NHS trust
- Two primary care groups
- Housing
- Regeneration
- Environment and health
- Social Services
- Chief Executive's department of the City Council
- Education department
- Early Years Partnership
- Voluntary Action Leicester
- Education Action Zone
- Life-Long Learning Partnership
- Sure Start Plus

The Leicester City multi-agency group has identified and developed four key themes for its first year.

1 *Effective provision*: education, prevention, clinical services, support to young parents. This will include further support for sex and relationships education both in schools and in non-school settings to increase the confidence and competence of staff in linking with those working in clinical settings. Other initiatives include involving community pharmacists in supplying emergency contraception, establishing a confidential telephone helpline to clinical services, exploring community-based condom provision, a focus on young men, and the further development of young people's advice and clinical services.

2 *Effective targeting of vulnerable young people*: this will include development of sex and relationships education for those at risk, especially young people who have been

excluded from school, those in residential and foster-care services, and Black and Asian young people, linking to other projects involving young people living in hostels or who are homeless.

3 *Linking strategies such as those described above and the media and communication strategy.*

4 *Effective engagement of young people in planning and practice*: the group will look for new opportunities to involve young people (e.g. via peer approaches).

The Tyne and Wear Health Action Zone has launched a major campaign on behalf of five multi-agency health partnerships. The 'Give a Little Love' campaign aims to make sexual healthcare more accessible for young people, with a freephone helpline and other initiatives, including opening new community clinics, extending existing clinic opening hours, working with schools, and the appointment of additional nurses and youth workers. A three-month publicity drive on the local radio and buses will promote the campaign.

The success of any partnership working depends on good relationships between partner organisations so that each shares a common understanding of what they are about and understands the roles played by all of the participants.

The Blakenall Health Start project has received Health Action Zone Innovations funding to pilot novel solutions in a deprived area as part of the regeneration of the community. The partners involved include Blakenall Local Committee, Community Association, Health Watch Group, Youth Council, North Primary Care Group and the Health Action Zone steering group. The partnership is

continued

supported by Walsall Health Authority, Walsall NHS Trusts, Social Services, Willenhall Police, Education and others. One of the project activities is to involve young men in innovative arts-based youth work with an emphasis on sexual health, teenage pregnancy and parenting, with a view to establishing a peer mentor programme for young men.[11]

Childline and teenage mentors

The following commentary by Steph Chambers reports her discussions with many of her contemporaries

Another way to seek help or advice is to ring Childline. It assures complete confidentiality and the phone number is free. This means that parents will not find out that their child has rung. It provides information and can deal with exactly what you want to know. Childline has counsellors on standby and offers a 24-hour service. It has proved extremely successful among the teenage population.

However, some teenagers would find it embarrassing to talk to Childline. They would find it difficult to talk to someone on the telephone even if they did not have to talk to them again. Some boys say that they would not feel able to talk to someone in this way and would find it very embarrassing. Girls may be able to talk to a counsellor on the phone more easily than boys because they generally find it easier to talk more openly.

Teenage mentors have been introduced at some schools, the idea being that younger members of the school can talk freely in front of older pupils. This is to save them the embarrassment of talking to teachers or other adults. They can trust fellow students who they look up to more than anyone else. They do not feel that they are being

continued

judged, and they therefore find it easier to talk. Pupils automatically assume that teachers have a preconceived idea about sexual behaviour and that they would never be able to agree with the type of behaviour that teenagers want to discuss, so why bother asking?

However, young people have mixed views about the usefulness of teenage mentors. Younger people would not necessarily receive the right advice from other teenagers, as in some cases the mentors are only 14 years old. Teenage mentors could give advice that they believe to be true when it is not, and most young teenagers would worry about seeing that particular mentor again at school every day. There is no definite guarantee of full confidentiality because it is very easy for pupils to talk among themselves, and the mentors might discuss the young teenager's problems or concerns with his or her friends. This applies especially in smaller schools where everyone knows everyone else, and also in the case of those who have brothers and sisters in the same school, especially if they are in the same year as the mentors.

Educational community-wide initiatives

Most of the 26 Health Action Zones have dedicated initiatives to reduce teenage pregnancy rates or established major programmes for improving the general health and well-being of young people. One such initiative in Manchester, Salford and Trafford is the 'Let's Get Serious' scheme which is establishing full-time mentoring to support young people with high levels of drug misuse, behavioural problems and poor educational performance. As these are all associated risk factors for teenage pregnancy these parallel initiatives should contribute to reducing teenage conception rates, too. Successful initiatives will require a co-ordinated approach involving all of the partner organisations and sectors that have a role in, or responsibility for, reducing the rate of teenage conceptions. One Health Action Zone-funded educational initiative that is focused on working with partners to find ways to influence teenagers' risk-taking behaviour through educational programmes is described in the box below.

Health Action Zone Innovations project to reduce teenage conceptions in Stoke-on-Trent

The high under-age teenage pregnancy rate in Stoke-on-Trent justified the successful bid to the NHS Executive's Health Action Zone Innovations Fund. Nearly 100 teenagers under 16 years of age become pregnant each year in the city.

The aim of the three-year project is to develop interactive educational programmes that make an impact on teenagers' behaviour such that they do not have unprotected sexual intercourse – that is, they either abstain from sexual intercourse, use contraception more effectively or use contraception more frequently and consistently.

- A teenage steering group drives the programme, facilitated by the project team. They will come up with the ideas and themes for the educational material destined for the teenage population across the city and beyond.
- Teenagers will frame their needs for contraception (education and services) and appropriate and effective information.
- Teenagers will develop educational material that meets their needs using their chosen media – paper based, electronic (informative and interactive), visual (video) or audio. The educational material will be used to create a culture of self-esteem and assertiveness, to inform others in the NHS, social services, voluntary sector and education of teenagers' needs, to provide sex education for teenagers, to provide accessible and up-to-date

continued

---

information about contraception, and to develop a network of school nurses or other appropriate mentors to offer electronic or telephone support.

- Specific multiprofessional education and training interventions based on the teenagers' ideas will enable doctors and nurses working within primary care groups, family planning service settings and others, to meet the contraceptive needs (education and services) of teenagers and their parents.
- Learner sets of multiprofessionals and representatives of the lay community should disseminate consistent messages and information within their organisations.
- The educational programme for teenagers will be trialled in young people's settings (e.g. local schools, teenage groups, youth clubs, work settings, town centre venues, etc.).
- Networking will take place with and through community development officers sited in youth settings (e.g. via youth workers who work alongside young people to teach them about the quality of relationships and motivate them to achieve and to feel more confident).

(Ruth Chambers, Project Leader,
Staffordshire University)

Access to contraceptive and advice services for young people

During 1998–99, about 1.2 million women and 80 000 men attended family planning clinics in England. About 20% of women who require family planning services attend family planning clinics, and the rest consult their GPs. Teenagers aged 16 to 19 years make most use of family planning clinics; 22% of women in this age group consulted a family planning clinic during 1998–99.[12]

General practices staffed by young female GPs or which have substantial practice nurse time are significantly less likely to have high teenage pregnancy rates compared to other practices, according to a study of 800 practices in the Trent region.[13] This study found that in practices with young female GPs, teenage pregnancy rates dropped to 75% of the expected level. In contrast, the availability of family planning clinics in the locality had no effect on the number of young girls who became pregnant.

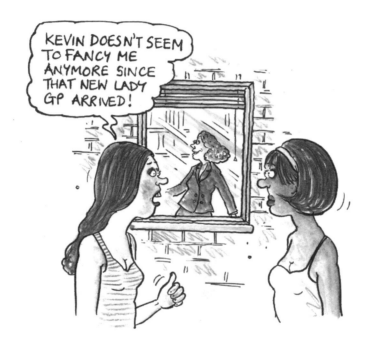

School nurse drop-in clinics sited in designated local general practices or community clinics have been established in North and Mid Staffordshire for several years. They are a popular way to bridge the gap between school and primary care, and their timing after school allows easy access for young people to obtain advice and help with contraception and relationship problems, as well as consulting about other lifestyle issues. Others elsewhere have called for more specialised teenage drop-in centres to which GPs can refer young people.

GPs and nurses in Paignton in Devon help to run a teenage information centre teenage advice centre (known as TIC TAC) at Paignton Community College during every lunchtime of the school term. A drugs and alcohol youth worker and a social worker are also available to give advice. Student representatives liaise between staff and students and give the health professionals feedback about the service on offer. The college is the only secondary school in the town, and is attended by 1700 pupils aged 11 to 18 years. In its first year there were 592 one-to-one consultations in the TIC TAC centre during the course of the 39-week academic year. Issues covered included sexuality, pregnancy advice, gambling, eating disorders, bereavement, smoking and stress.[14]

The Cornwall initiative described earlier aims to extend access on a community-wide basis, but many general practices have set up special initiatives to encourage the young people in their patient populations to take a pro-active approach to contraception and other lifestyle issues, as the examples below demonstrate.

The Royal College of General Practitioners (RCGP)/ Brook training kit enables general practices to think through four scenarios illustrating difficult situations where confidentiality issues arise. The resource enables practice teams to discuss and agree their policies on confidentiality for young teenagers. It then encourages them to advertise their policy clearly in the practice leaflet, advising teenagers that they can go for contraceptive help and advice to any other practice, and providing contact details of doctors nearby who would be happy to see them.[15]

Students at Seaford Head Community College near Eastbourne wrote a colourful leaflet that comes with a card for teenagers to complete and hand to receptionists to make a prompt confidential appointment to see a doctor – either their own general practitioner or any other GP at two participating Seaford practices.[16]

One practice that advertised the availability of its family planning services to patients in general from outside its practice trebled its income from contraceptive services. The clinic runs from 4.30 p.m. to 7.00 p.m. for one evening a week, and the practice nurse, health visitor and GP see about 25 patients of all ages during a session.[17]

A five-partner practice in Stafford with a patient list size of 9200 has been running a successful teenage health clinic for several years. Teenagers are invited to call in for a chat about health issues such as smoking, alcohol, diet, drugs, contraception and relationship problems at home or at school. The poster advertising the service emphasises that the young person can expect confidential advice from a health visitor, practice nurse or doctor, and may just drop in or make an appointment between 4 and 6 p.m. on the first and third Thursday of every month. The clinic sees an average of 52% of the teenage patient population of the practice during their sixteenth year – boys as well as girls. The practice sends out unsolicited appointments – booked for 20 minutes – offering to swap the time if it is not convenient. They advertise the service in all of the local high schools and youth and social clubs.

Easy access to emergency contraception is very important for teenagers whose sexual activity may be unplanned and sporadic. There is widespread public and professional misunderstanding of emergency contraception, including criteria for appropriate use, the options available, the timing, the location of services, etc.[5] For instance, many health professionals are unaware that an intra-uterine device may be offered to a nulliparous teenager as emergency contraception and fitted up to five days after the expected day of ovulation.

> The Dales Primary Care Group in Durham is investing £5000 in an initiative that encourages GPs to advertise their services to teenagers who are registered at other practices. They have agreed to see teenagers without appointments or during school lunch hours. The participating GPs have free condoms to distribute.[18]

A variety of services are being piloted to improve both knowledge of what is available and the ease with which the contraceptives can be obtained (e.g. in community pharmacies as described below).

Community pharmacists

Community pharmacists are liaising with general medical practitioners in some Health Action Zones and some primary care groups in several pilot sites in the UK, to provide the emergency contraceptive pill as a pharmacy medicine over the counter, rather than it being available by prescription only. The Committee on Safety of Medicines has recommended that women aged 16 years or over can safely receive the progesterone-only emergency contraceptive (levonorgestrel 0.75 mg as Levonelle-2) without seeing a doctor. A randomised controlled trial of emergency contraception kept at home or obtained from a doctor showed no difference in the proportion of women in the two groups who used emergency contraception twice or more during the year of the study, and emergency contraception was almost always used correctly.[19]

A 14-year-old girl's attempts to seek emergency contraception

The following commentary tracks Steph Chambers as she tries to seek emergency contraceptive help

I thought that the best way to find out where teenagers were missing out was to pretend that I was in need of starting the pill or even obtaining the emergency contraceptive pill. I asked myself how I would go about finding my nearest family planning clinic.

My first step was to go and find the Yellow Pages, which my family happens to have, but there are many teenagers who would not be able to get their hands on this resource. I looked up 'Family Planning Clinics' to find adverts that did not seem to help me find out the whereabouts or the name of the local family planning clinic in my area. The adverts that were there were for national centres. This put me off ringing because it seemed as if it was set up for people with very important problems, and all I wanted was to talk to someone local and find out the area where the nearest family planning clinic was situated.

Luckily, I saw the entry 'see Clinics', so I looked up this section. I was faced with a range of clinics, each with various telephone numbers. This seemed more promising, and I thought that I was going to be able to find it easily. However, I was then confused because I could not tell the difference between sports clinics, etc. and family planning clinics. I was unsure about this, and was disinclined to pick one and call and just hope for the best.

I then thought that I would go to another type of resource and find the phone book. Again many teenage girls would not have one readily available. I looked up 'Family Planning Clinics,' which proved to be reasonably easy, and I found a few. However, there were not many,

continued

and the nearest one to me seemed to be about 10 or 15 minutes' car travelling time away. This did not seem right, but if I really was in that situation then I would have just telephoned.

I glanced down to what appeared to be the next topic. It was only then that I realised that it was not a new topic at all but a continuation of the list of clinics. The only reason why I realised this was because I recognised one of the names of a clinic that I had come across before. It had confused and misled me because what seemed to me to be a new topic was actually just a new sub-heading – 'First Community Trust'. It began with the letter 'f' like the rest of the topics in this section of the phone book, and was like a new title. I did not know what 'First Community Trust' meant, and it should have been more clearly marked. The clinics that were listed had no opening times shown.

I looked to see if there was any other type of information in any other sections of the phone book, and I discovered that there were even more Family Planning Clinics under 'Health'. The thing that puzzled me was why there were nearly four times as many clinics listed there and they still had no opening times shown next to them.

How can teenagers find information effectively if the only resource they have is too difficult to follow, difficult to use, and it misleads and confuses them? The Yellow Pages should have clear headings indicating what each clinic is offering, rather than signposting the reader to more information on other pages. The entries about clinics should state whether there is any more information available on other pages, and should give the relevant page numbers and subjects.

Therefore if I was in that situation and I could not find a family planning centre near to me, would I have bothered travelling miles to another one? The answer is no!

Teenagers do prefer anonymity when they are obtaining contraceptives. Condom vending machines in public toilets are a popular choice, rather than collecting supplies from a school nurse.[20]

Family planning clinics

The following commentary by Steph Chambers describes what her contemporaries have told her

Not many teenagers know about family planning clinics. Only a few would know where their nearest family planning clinic was in relation to where they lived, and even if they did, fewer still would know the opening hours of the clinic.

Family planning clinics should advertise their services at places that are widely frequented by teenagers, such as youth clubs and schools, and should also raise awareness about what they offer.

A family planning clinic offers free contraception. It is one of the only places to do so, and teenagers need to have the knowledge necessary to take advantage of the service offered by the clinic.

You can ask questions and receive the relevant information in return, and all consultations are confidential. There is a range of leaflets (to which you can help yourself) that also offer information on different subjects. Family planning clinics do have the potential to become an effective service with a higher percentage of teenagers attending, but at present knowledge of their existence is too reliant on word of mouth.

Effective methods of reducing rates of teenage pregnancy – workshop conclusions

Nearly 50 primary care professionals, schoolteachers, community development officers, school nurses, health promotion facilitators, social workers and others working in the voluntary sector came together to focus on effective ways to reduce the teenage pregnancy rate in the North Staffordshire district. The outcomes of the initial discussions were circulated after the event so that the participants could add any extra ideas and vote for those which they thought were most likely to be effective. Table 2.1 lists the most popular ideas for initiatives that should be adopted or extended.

A novel approach by the Wolverhampton Wanderers football club provides an example of some of the ideas generated from the workshop for focusing on teenage boys and young men in more imaginative ways. The government has given the football club £230 000 to provide local boys with a football coaching programme together with sessions for discussing the risks of unprotected sex. Another male-targeted programme in Buckinghamshire is being run in a general practice where teenage sex education is highlighted in discussions at Fathers and Sons evenings. [21]

Table 2.1: Workshop participants' suggestions for ways to reduce teenage pregnancy rates across the district (n = 48 participants including health professionals, teachers, community development workers, youth workers, strategists and academics)

Ideas from participants	n
Action that the health service might take	48
Young people's advice and contraception clinics (confidential, convenient times, new settings)	32
Condoms should be available free of charge from GP practices, not just family planning clinics	31
Increase access to family planning/condoms, etc.	30
Improve access to emergency contraception	29
School nurses should be allowed to supply the morning-after pill	25
More school nurses should be involved in drop-in contraceptive and advice services	25
Confidentiality policies should be widely advertised in the NHS – in general practices, family planning clinics, etc.	22

Table 2.1: continued

Ideas from participants	n
Action that the health service might take (continued)	
Contraceptive information should be available closer to the people who want it (e.g. in clinics, schools)	22
Find a new name for family planning	20
Out-of-school setting for school nurse advice	20
Dispel the stigma of attending a family planning clinic	20
Relationships should be built with school nurses, rolling programmes with nurses	20
NHS should build relationships with schools	15
Male GPs should talk to boys in schools	14
NHS work with voluntary sector organisations	9
Practical approaches in schools/youth settings	
Access to condoms in schools and other young people-friendly environments	25
Teenage mentors to advise and support younger pupils	18
Educational approaches to young people	
Educate young people about sexual health as part of personal health and social education at school	31
Accept that risk taking will always occur, and concentrate on building self-esteem, assertiveness and social skills	31
Create a culture change – reduce peer pressure and educate about the impact of parenting	27
Build the confidence/self-esteem of young women	24
Innovative publicity about contraception/not getting pregnant	22
Peer education via drama/video; young people making videos themselves	21
Internet websites on sexual health produced by schools for schools	21
Overcome the problem of other school education impeding effective sexual health education	17
Explore real-life experiences	16
Have a parents' evening on reducing teenage pregnancy rates and input to curriculum	15
Peer teaching (e.g. at youth clubs)	14

Table 2.1: continued

Ideas from participants	n
Educational approaches to young people (continued)	
Overcome barriers (and beliefs that teaching is for teachers, not nurses)	12
Highlight performance of the school/college in preventing teenage pregnancy, but make allowance for type of young population in individual schools	12
Target Catholic schools – encourage openness, set up advice centres	11
Educational approaches to staff	
Train teachers, school nurses and youth workers in how to talk about sex and relationships, so that everyone is prepared for situations that come their way	31
Educate staff in contact with young people to adopt sensitive attitudes	26
Ensure all professionals have a standard set of information to give (about contraception, sex, relationships) via newsletters or learning package	16
Accept that we all (professionals and young people alike) have hang-ups about sex	11
Practical support to young people	
'Drop-ins' at schools before or after school lunch-breaks	25
Build relationships with youth workers	17
Overcome cultural barriers (e.g. promote teenage sexual health in youth clubs)	12
Homestart (mother-and-baby group)	11
Good practice in communicating messages	
Images and not necessarily words	12
User-friendly educational and communication materials	24
Understandable language	21
Drama workshops	14
Avoid the present situation where users of family planning clinics get 'labelled'	13
Use a problem page of a local magazine	12
Work with the press and the media (e.g. with those producing magazines for boys)	12

Table 2.1: continued

Ideas from participants	n
Good practice in communicating messages (continued)	
Video approach	10
Hold separate meetings for young men and women	10
District-wide or partnership approach	
Appropriate venue in youth clubs for contraceptive advice clinics	29
Target boys more effectively in future; focus on young men	25
Arrange for young parents to talk to young people	24
Bring contraceptive and advice services nearer to areas where people live	21
Target younger age groups	19
Change the culture (open-minded countries have reduced young pregnancy rates)	18
Put on a roadshow of some sort to provide information/education (e.g. bus)	18
Promote collaboration/partnerships between professionals responsible for young	17
Advertise condoms in innovative ways (e.g. with a company like adidas)	16
Take resources out to clients	14
Promote sexual health, etc. via recorded information (e.g. local radio station)	14
Encourage pilot projects such as the Young Carers Project	11
Punish 'adult' men who have sex with under-age girls	8
Give young people incentives not to get pregnant, such as money 'vouchers'	3

References

1   Aggleton P, Oliver C and Rivers K (1998) *Reducing the Rate of Teenage Conceptions: the implications of research into young people, sex, sexuality and relationships.* Health Education Authority, London.

2   NHS Centre for Reviews and Dissemination (1997) Preventing and reducing the adverse effects of unintended teenage pregnancies. *Effective Health Care Bull.* **3**: 1–12.

3   Ashton J (1994) Teenage pregnancy – common sense begins to pay off at last. *Update.* **15 Nov**: 567–8.

4   Pedrazzini A, McGowan H and Johanson R (2000) The trouble with sex – it always gets in the way. An evaluation of a peer-produced teenage pregnancy video. *Br J Fam Plan.* **26**(3): 131–5.

5   Hughes K (1999) *Reducing the Rate of Teenage Conceptions. Young People's Experiences of Relationships, Sex and Early Parenthood: Qualitative Research.* Health Education Authority, London.

6   Department of Health (1999) *Teenage Pregnancy.* Social Exclusion Unit, Department of Health, London.

7   Oakley A, Fullerton D, Holland J *et al.* (1995) Sexual health education interventions for young people: a methodological review. *BMJ.* **310**: 158–62.

8   Meyrick J and Swann C (1998) *Reducing the Rate of Teenage Conceptions. An Overview of the Effectiveness of Interventions and Programmes Aimed at Reducing Unintended Conceptions in Young People.* Health Education Authority, London.

9   Chief Medical Officer (2000) *Local Teenage Pregnancy Co-ordinators Appointed.* Chief Medical Officer's Update 26. Department of Health, London.

10 Tilbury J (2000) *Increasing Young People's Access to Primary Care Sexual Services. A HAZ Fellowship Application.* Gunnislake, Cornwall.

11 Walsall Health Partnership (1999) *HAZ Innovations Fund Blakenall Health Start.* Walsall Health Authority, Walsall.

12 Department of Health (1999) *NHS Contraceptive Services, England: 1998–99.* Department of Health, London.

13 Hippisley-Cox J, Allen J, Pringle M *et al.* (2000) The associations between general practice characteristics and teenage pregnancy rates: cross-sectional survey in Trent, 1994 to 1997. *BMJ.* **320**: 842–6.

14 Bridge J (2000) How we set up an advice service in a local school. *GP News*. **4 Feb**: 69.

15 Royal College of General Practitioners/Brook Advisory Centres (2000) *Confidentiality and Young People. Improving Teenagers' Uptake of Health Advice: a toolkit for general practices and primary care groups/trusts*. RCGP/Brook Advisory Centres in conjunction with the RCN, BMA, DoH, MDU, London.

16 Shears M (2000) GP helps teenagers to make access easier. *Pulse*. **60**(22): 1.

17 Law K (2000) GPs' contraception clinic is major hit. *Pulse*. **29 April**: 8.

18 Findlay S (2000) Free condoms to avert teenage pregnancy. *GP News*. **16 June**: 14.

19 Glasier A and Baird D (1998) The effects of self-administered emergency contraception. *NEJM*. **339**: 1–4.

20 Kaul S (1993) Teenagers, sex and risk-taking. *BMJ*. **307**: 683 (letter).

21 Anon (2000) The birds, the bees and the boys. *Good Housekeeping*. **July**: 175.

CHAPTER 3

Clinical governance – using clinical governance to tackle teenage pregnancy rates and improve access to and availability of contraceptive services for young people

Clinical governance is about finding ways to 'implement care that works in an environment in which clinical effectiveness can flourish by establishing a facilitatory culture'.[1] The increasing emphasis on team-based learning that includes everyone – whether they are a doctor, a nurse, a manager or a provider of non-clinical support – should help to deliver a more co-ordinated approach across primary healthcare to reducing teenage conception rates. Clinical governance will underpin individuals' and team-based professional development plans, which should in turn link into the business and development plans of their primary care group (PCG)/trust (PCT) and the district as a whole (see Figure 3.1). This should encourage linkages and joint working between primary care and the non-health sector, NHS trusts and community programmes. The shared goal of halving conception rates in those under 18 years of age by the year 2010 should narrow the

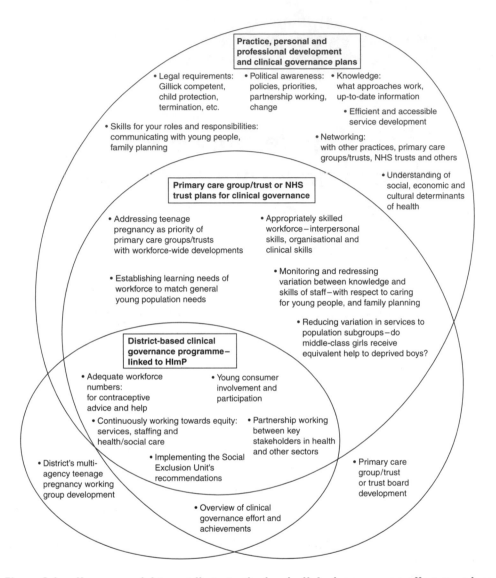

Figure 3.1: How you might contribute to the local clinical governance effort to reduce teenage conception rates in your current post. Note that the topics given as priority areas for development are examples and are not intended to constitute comprehensive lists.

focus of direction of continuing professional development to meet the young population's health needs.

Clinical governance is concerned with combining quality improvement and accountability to:

- sustain quality improvements
- minimise inequalities in the health of different subgroups of the population
- reduce variations in healthcare services
- define standards
- demonstrate achievements.

Minimising inequalities is at the heart of clinical governance. There are two aspects:

- *inequalities in healthcare*: variations in access, service provision or standards of care and discrimination on the grounds of age, gender, ethnicity, sexuality, disability, etc.
- *inequalities in people's health*: influenced both by risky lifestyles and by social determinants of health, such as poor housing, low income and lack of transport.

This approach to inequalities is relevant to the culture needed to establish the types of multi-faceted interventions that were described in Chapters 1 and 2, which have the potential to reduce teenage conception rates.

The components of clinical governance are not new. However, bringing them together under the banner of clinical governance and introducing more explicit accountability for performance is a new style of working.[2]

We have described the 14 themes of a quality healthcare service that constitute clinical governance in detail elsewhere.[2] The components and ideas with regard to what you might do as part of your clinical governance programme are as follows.

Establishing a learning culture

You might convene an educational session in your practice for your primary healthcare team with the district's teenage pregnancy co-ordinator or sexual health promotion facilitator, and invite local school nurses or others from outside the practice who might be interested. You might all gain more insight into young men's needs, and brush up on best practice (e.g. with emergency contraception). It is not only doctors who need to know more about new methods such as progesterone-only emergency contraception pills. Discuss as a practice team how to make the surgery more 'teenager friendly' (e.g. consider the appearance of the waiting-room or the consultation rooms, and the systems and procedures that are used).

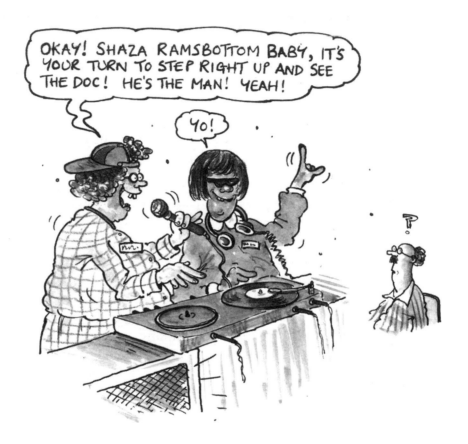

Managing resources and services

The receptionists should be flexible about accommodating young people's requests for help, and must be sensitive to their shyly asking for immediate consultations. Your contraceptive services for young people should be easily accessible and readily available. Are staff available when they are needed? Could their availability be changed to meet the needs? Are doctors and staff suitably qualified for the work they do in looking after young people's sexual health or would more training improve your services (e.g. in fitting emergency intra-uterine devices)? All members of the practice or clinic team should know the details of other advice and support services in the neighbourhood.

> The factors that were blocking easy access to consultations with GPs in one study of 15- to 16-year-old adolescents were lack of trust in confidentiality, lack of staff friendliness, and delay in appointments.[3]

Advertise the fact that contraception is available and that treatment is confidential, and appeal to boys as well as girls. Try to link into a free condom distribution scheme. You could also consider running a dedicated young person's clinic in the practice at times that are convenient for young people.

Establishing a research and development culture

Find out what young people want and how best to engage them and make an impact on their behaviour. Search the literature for examples of best practice. Should you undertake your own study of an aspect of contraceptive care for young people? Is there a member of staff whose job is to disseminate knowledge of changes in clinical management or new guidelines?

Reliable and accurate data

Be aware of how many young people are attending for contraception and whether there are clusters of unplanned pregnancies in particular areas. Improve your data recording and plan who will be involved in this. Do you all record data in such a way that you can easily find out how many teenagers you saw for emergency contraception last year?

Evidence-based practice and policy

A clinical update meeting might focus on the 'best' ways to explain risk to young people. Incorporate the evidence into improved ways of working. Do you have evidence-based nurse protocols that enhance teamworking?

Confidentiality

Everyone should know and understand the rules for preserving confidentiality in relation to patients under 16 years of age. Many young people do not attend GP surgeries because they fear that their details will not remain confidential. If the last consultation is displayed on your computer screen, how do you prevent a person accompanying a teenager (e.g. a parent) from seeing that information on the screen next time they attend?

Health gain

There are direct health gains for the young person, their parents and the unborn child (e.g. avoiding poverty and low birthweight babies). Include learning about the social, economic and cultural determinants of health in your practice, personal and professional development plan. Does everyone involved in the provision of contraception in your practice (including GPs, nurses and receptionists) know the health risks when very young teenagers become pregnant? Do the teenagers themselves know these risks?

Coherent team

Partnership working will lead to those in the NHS working more closely with anti-poverty workers in the local council, social workers, children in care, schools, the general public, the media and press, and social and leisure organisations. You will have to create and sustain partnerships, and you need to plan how to do that. Good communication with all staff involved and an understanding of each other's roles and responsibilities will be vital in any initiative to reduce teenage pregnancy rates when different professionals are working together from their own organisations.

Practice staff should know where else young people can obtain emergency contraception if your GPs are not available or if your practice is unable to help. These sources of contraception would include young people's family planning clinics, condom vending machines, other more willing GPs, etc.

> Many young people do not know where to find family planning clinics or how to access them.[4]

Audit and evaluation

Monitor how many young people consult for contraception. Do you know how this figure compares with those for other practices? Plan and execute improvements in services. Health professionals can use audit to check that they are providing good-quality contraceptive services to the majority of their patients.[5] If claims for contraceptive services in a practice are low, do the doctors or practice nurses need more training in sexual health and contraception so that they can be more proactive and effective? Are the receptionists sensitive to the needs of patients who are seeking contraceptive care?

Meaningful involvement of patients and the public

Establish how a young person who is unfamiliar with the workings of your practice would access emergency contraception. You could ask a young patient to give you their perspectives about the barriers, in much the same way that Steph did in Chapter 2. Try introducing a card system[6] (whereby young girls who need emergency contraception show a card to the receptionist) to avoid delay. Make sure that patients know the practice is interested in and receptive to their needs.

Improve staff expertise in engaging individual young people in making decisions and informed choices. Seek young people's input or exchange information about the services you provide (e.g. through a focus group discussion with teenagers). If you do not know much about meaningful involvement, incorporate that learning into your practice, personal and professional development plan.

Health promotion

Focus on health promotion messages about safe sex whenever a young person consults you for emergency contraception (the basic messages are safe from pregnancy, safe from infection and safe from coercion). Establish a good rapport in the emergency situation, and the young person will then be more likely to return for more routine care when you can discuss the health risks associated with smoking and excessive alcohol and substance abuse. Learn more about the long-term effects of sexual infection (e.g. increased rates of infertility resulting from infection with chlamydia). Learn about the association between alcohol and drug misuse and unwanted pregnancy, and how to motivate teenagers to resist or reduce risky behaviour.

Make sure that your health promotion literature is available in all the languages of your patient population. For instance, the manufacturers of the progesterone depot injection produce patient information leaflets in English, Greek, Bengali, Hindi, Chinese, Punjabi, Urdu, Gujarati and Turkish.

Risk management

Concentrate on controlling the most common sources of risk in primary care, namely lack of continuity of care, poor communication, and informing virgins about emergency contraception. Work with teachers and parents to give them accurate information about contraception which they in turn can relay to young people, and debunk myths that might tempt young people to take unnecessary risks.

Accountability and performance

Demonstrate the standards of services that you provide and the care for which you are accountable, both as individual practitioners and for the practice as a whole. Evaluate your performance and any changes.

Core requirements

Deliver education and training both in-house and through external courses so that your staff are competent and their skill mix is appropriate for your local circumstances and population needs. Practice nurses are often perceived by young people as more approachable and less threatening than doctors. Look at the skills, knowledge and attitudes of all members of your staff. You should also review your environment. Does it seem comfortable, welcoming and safe?

Provide 'seamless' contraceptive services within a district

Complement good access to readily available contraceptive services in general practices and family planning clinics with easy referral to secondary care when obstetric and gynaecological care is appropriate (e.g. the antenatal care of pregnant teenagers or terminations for those young people who do not wish to continue with their pregnancies). Link school nurses in as part of the integrated provision of contraceptive services in your district.

The need for good counselling and support for pregnant teenagers is discussed in Chapter 7.

The NHS funded 73% of all abortions in England and Wales in 1997. Provision varies widely between areas, with some funding over 90% and some less than 50%.[7] Even in areas where abortion is funded, the woman may have to travel long distances to contracted-out services in another area. Charitable or private agencies may be the only option in some areas, especially if there has been a delay and the pregnancy is over 12 weeks gestation. This is an area for action to remove 'postcode' inequalities and improve access for all, but especially for the young and the poor, who are particularly disadvantaged by the present system.

Following concerns about delays for termination of pregnancy and conflicts between provision for gynaecology and terminations, a one-stop clinic was set up by a family planning service,[8] which is open each lunch time Monday to Friday. Two part-time clerks book the referrals in and make sure that all of the relevant paperwork is done. A family planning-trained nurse and doctor see the patients for counselling, examination, swabs and blood samples. If the patient is unsure about what to do,

continued

she can also see a specialist counsellor. An appointment for admission to the day unit is made within the next few days. Family planning doctors with special training perform the termination in the day theatre, and most women are discharged four to five hours later. Back-up for any complications is provided by the general gynaecological service. The service offers a 100% district-wide service for first-trimester abortions. Second-trimester abortions are worked up in the same way, but the small number of procedures are performed in a more specialised unit provided by the charitable organisation known as the British Pregnancy Advisory Service (BPAS). Close liaison with family planning services provides good follow-up and advice on future contraception.

In many areas, women presenting for termination face uncertain waiting times and resentment by medical and nursing staff who would rather be dealing with the waiting-list of serious gynaecological procedures. Women may be admitted to general gynaecological wards where they have to mix with other patients who may be being investigated for infertility. There may be no follow-up contraceptive advice or supplies given before the patient leaves the unit, due to pressure of work or lack of foresight.

The British Pregnancy Advisory Service (BPAS) aims to offer women an assessment appointment within five days of initial contact and, if appropriate, an abortion procedure within seven days of assessment. They offer care under an NHS agency arrangement as well as a private service. Revised guidelines relating to the provision of abortion by the BPAS have allowed the service to improve patient choice and confidentiality by discharging patients

continued

when they are medically fit to travel, rather than waiting until a fixed time, and terminations are carried out up to 19 weeks rather than up to the previous limit of 14 weeks gestation.

References

1   Chambers R and Wall D (1999) *Teaching Made Easy: a manual for health professionals*. Radcliffe Medical Press, Oxford.

2   Chambers R and Wakley G (2000) *Making Clinical Governance Work for You*. Radcliffe Medical Press, Oxford.

3   Donovan C, Mellanby A, Jacobson L *et al.* (1997) Teenagers' views on the general practice consultation and provision of contraception. *Br J Gen Pract*. **47**: 715–18.

4   Francome C and Walsh J (1995) *Young Teenage Pregnancy*. Middlesex University and the Family Planning Association, Middlesex.

5   Rowlands S (1997) *Managing Family Planning in General Practice*. Radcliffe Medical Press, Oxford.

6   Family Planning Association (1999) *Emergency Contraception Pack*. This contains posters, leaflets and 'credit cards' for requesting emergency contraception, and is available from CES at the Family Planning Association, 2–12 Pentonville Road, London N1 9FP.

7   Abortion Law Reform Association (1997) *A Report on NHS Abortion Services*. Abortion Law Reform Association, London.

8   Randall S (1996) Provision of a district abortion service by a community family planning service. *Br J Fam Plan*. **21**: 152.

CHAPTER 4

Reaching young people – meaningful involvement

Sharing information – patient-held records

You may need to discuss explicitly with the patient what information will be passed on to other members of the team. Patient-held records have been shown to ensure that everyone, including the patient, knows what information is in the public domain. Some general practices have experimented with patient-held record cards for contraception. Although at first sight this might seem an ideal way of involving the user, where would a teenager actually keep a health record private, and would they remember to bring it with them to every consultation about their health or sexual needs? Evaluation is clearly needed!

Barriers in communication

An American omnibus survey of teenagers and parents of teenagers in 1998 explored what respondents thought was the 'greatest barrier to effective communication between parents and teens on sex and relationships'.[1] The most common blocks to communication were thought to be that 'most teenagers think they know it all already' (32% of parents) and 'teenagers

are not comfortable hearing from their parents about sex'
(39% of teenagers and 30% of parents). Other frequently
mentioned blocks to communication were that 'parents are not
comfortable talking to their kids about sex' (24% of parents
and 17% of teenagers), 'teens don't want to hear from their
parents about sex' (19% of parents), 'parents are too judgemental' (14% of teenagers) and 'parents don't know what to
say' (9% of parents).

More openness about sex would lead to young people being
able to talk more freely and honestly with their parents. In The
Netherlands there is more openness about sex within the
home, as well as early and consistent sex education in schools.
The culture in The Netherlands is characterised by young
people being able to:

- maintain friendships and discuss problems with both sexes
- communicate effectively with a sexual partner or potential
  partner
- negotiate use of contraception
- think about, plan and use safer sex practices
- discuss the meaning and importance of sex within a relationship.[2]

Getting the language right

Health professionals and teachers should use the same
language that young people use when talking about sex on a
one-to-one basis or teaching in school. If the adult does have to
use professional language, they should explain what the
technical terms mean.

User involvement and consultation of the young public

Guidelines for health authorities and local authorities on tackling teenage pregnancy put 'involving young people' as a plank

of a local strategy to audit the 'effectiveness of services and seek their views on future service design'.[3] If future services are to be 'attractive to teenagers and offer what they value most', as well as responding to 'patterns of needs for the different ethnic communities', then user involvement and consultation of the young public will be necessary components in planning any contraceptive and sexual health services for young people.

> The government has tried to gauge young people's views in order to compile the report *Listen Up*, which has been published jointly by the Home Office and the Cabinet Office. This report concludes that 'young women often do what they think men want, and feel unable to express their own needs and preferences'. To obtain this type of qualitative material from a diverse group of young people, the researchers convened discussion groups, ran a survey on the Internet and arranged for the politicians to meet young people in a city-centre nightclub.[4]

If an exercise designed to seek people's opinions is to be meaningful, it must involve people who represent that section of the population which the consultation concerns. People in groups that are difficult to reach, such as young people, will be most unlikely to come forward and express their views unless you use an intermediary such as a youth worker or another young person. Many consultations currently involve the most accessible people, who are not necessarily representative of the community with whom you want to engage. Although everyone's views are important, a wide range of other young people's opinions are needed as well, if the consultation is to be anything more than a token activity. You will have to set up systems to actively seek out and involve young people. Moreover, if you do manage to reach young people, it is important not to get to know them too well or use them too often, as your relationship with them will then become too close and cosy and they will no longer be truly representative of other teenagers.[5]

One practice in Wales attempted to engage teenage mothers in a rapid participatory appraisal of contraceptive services in the practice, in order to identify barriers to accessing advice and help. The project plan was to identify the 'community of interest' – in this case the 29 teenagers who had given birth in the previous three years, current pregnant teenagers and key individuals who might have constructive views on teenage pregnancy. The teenagers were approached opportunistically or by telephone, and tracking them down proved very difficult. In total, 42 of the identified 49 subjects were identified to find out what they thought of the services, and a meeting of all subjects was then convened to consider the group's views on what changes to services were most important and then to make those changes in practice. There was considerable apathy (only 10 of the 42 subjects who were interviewed attended the group feedback meeting). The practice is now willing to share its expertise in rapid participatory appraisal with others in its local health group.[6]

Getting a community-wide initiative off the ground

One good example of the power of a community-wide approach in Sweden has involved skilling and empowering a nucleus of 'experts' within a community, and letting the information and expertise spread 'like rings on the water'. The initiative promoting positive sexual health and the prevention of unwanted teenage pregnancy and infection by sexually transmitted diseases has been successfully implemented in more than half of Sweden. The community-wide initiatives aim to break down barriers between generations, increase sexual choice and make an impact on young people's sexual behaviour. The main thrust is through intensive residential workshops for key opinion-formers, decision-makers, role models, teachers, other professionals and counsellors of young people. Workshops held throughout a county involve people in the towns and schools of neighbourhoods. The participants become 'resource persons' for the programme initiatives, with knowledge and skills rippling out through the community from the centre. Teenagers visit community clinics to familiarise themselves with the services that are available there, discussions encourage the concept of a couple taking joint responsibility for contraception, and the media help to promote city-wide debates about the nature of sexuality and the community response. As a result teenage conception rates have fallen by 40% and the incidence of sexually transmitted diseases has shown a similar decline.[7]

References

1 National Campaign to Prevent Teen Pregnancy (1998) *National Omnibus Survey*. National Campaign to Prevent Teen Pregnancy, Washington, DC.

2 Aggleton P, Oliver C and Rivers K (1998) *Reducing the Rate of Teenage Conceptions – the Implications of Research into Young People, Sex, Sexuality and Relationships*. Health Education Authority, London.

3 Hamlyn C (2000) *Tackling Teenage Pregnancy: action for health authorities and local authorities*. Teenage Pregnancy Unit, Department of Health, London.

4 Frean A (2000) Girl Power: girls still lack the power to say no. *The Times*. **12 April**: 12.

5 Chambers R (2000) *Involving Patients and the Public: how to do it better*. Radcliffe Medical Press, Oxford.

6 Morgan R (2000) Did primary care advice really fail our pregnant teenagers? *Primary Care Rep*. **April**: 38–41.

7 Ashton J (1989) True story: the Liverpool project to reduce teenage pregnancy. *Br J Fam Plan*. **15**: 46–51.

CHAPTER 5

Confidentiality and young people's concerns

Teenagers' views

Sexual activity is regarded as private, and concerns about confidentiality often deter young people from seeking help. As many as a quarter of adolescents[1] believe that their parents will be informed about their consultations with general practices.

> Many teenagers who attend young people's clinics do not consent to information about their consultation being passed on to their own GP, as they do not believe that the information will be kept confidential. They also have doubts about clinics – quite a sizeable minority of teenagers give false names or dates of birth or refuse to give their addresses. This creates problems when they attend the next time, as they are sure that they have been before, but no notes in their (real) name can be found. It is even more confusing if they have given the name of a friend as their own – especially when that friend also attends!

Concerns about confidentiality decrease the more often the teenager consults without their parents and their experience shows that deliberate breaches of confidentiality are unlikely.

A randomised controlled trial demonstrated that the doctor providing information about confidentiality[2] could increase the willingness of adolescents to attend, disclose sensitive information and be honest.

Concerns about confidentiality at general practice surgeries may include fears of being seen there by relatives or other people who know the teenager concerned. Confidentiality of consultations about contraception is known to be a major source of anxiety for teenagers.[3,4,5] A confidentiality toolkit has been produced by the RCGP and Brook Advisory Centres.[5]

Confidentiality and young people

Nurses and doctors are bound by their professional conduct requirements, and confidentiality can only be breached under certain specified circumstances. Young people under the age of 16 years have the same rights to confidentiality as other patients. The younger the person, the more care is needed to assess the level of understanding to ensure that the patient understands the consequences of any proposed action.

The 'Fraser Guidelines' (also known as the Gillick Guidelines) were drawn up after Lord Fraser's judgement following the House of Lords ruling in the case of *Victoria Gillick v West Norfolk and Wisbech Health Authority*. Lord Fraser stated in 1985 that a doctor could give contraceptive advice or treatment to a person under 16-years-old without parental consent, provided that the doctor is satisfied that:

- the young person will understand the advice
- they cannot be persuaded to tell their parents or allow the doctor to tell them that they are seeking contraceptive advice
- they are likely to begin or continue to have unprotected sex with or without contraceptive treatment

continued

> - their physical or mental health is likely to suffer unless they receive contraceptive advice or treatment
> - it is in the young person's best interest to give them contraceptive advice or treatment.

If a young person fulfils these conditions he or she is popularly referred to as being 'Gillick competent'.

The Department of Health have recently issued new guidance for health professionals about confidentiality for under 16-year-olds as part of its new Sexual Health Strategy.[6] This replaces the 1986 post-Gillick guidance (*see* Chapter 6).

Principles of confidentiality in healthcare

The principle of confidentiality is basic to the practice of healthcare. Patients attend for healthcare in the belief that the information that they supply, or which is found out about them during investigation or treatment, will be kept private.

Health professionals are responsible to patients with whom they are in a professional relationship for the confidentiality and security of any information obtained about them. They must preserve privacy about all that they know. The fundamental principle is that they must not use or disclose any confidential information obtained in the course of their clinical work, other than for the clinical care of the patient to whom that information relates.

The only exceptions to the above occur if:

- the patient consents
- it is in the patient's own interest that information should be disclosed, but it is either impossible, or medically undesirable in the patient's own interest, to seek the patient's consent
- the law requires (and does not merely permit) the health professional to disclose the information

- the health professional agrees that disclosure is necessary to safeguard national security
- the disclosure is necessary to prevent a serious risk to public health
- the disclosure is needed for the purposes of medical research in certain circumstances.

Health professionals must be able to justify any decision to disclose information without consent. If they are in any doubt about this, they should consult their professional bodies and colleagues.

Consent to disclosure

Information given to a health professional remains the property of the patient. In general, consent is assumed for the *necessary* sharing of information with other professionals involved with the care of the patient for that episode of care and, where essential, for continuing care. Beyond this, informed consent must be obtained.

The consent is only valid if the patient fully understands the nature and consequences of disclosure. If consent is given, the health worker is responsible for limiting the disclosure to that information for which informed consent has been obtained. If you pass on information (with consent) to a non-professional organisation or person, you must ensure that the confidential nature of the information is understood (e.g. marked 'private and confidential').

The development of modern information technology and the increasing amount of multidisciplinary teamwork in patient care make confidentiality difficult to uphold. You should be aware that patients often underestimate the amount of information sharing that occurs. Patients' expectations and attitudes show considerable divergence from accepted practice. Many of them feel that administrative and secretarial staff should not have access to their medical records. Some patients have reservations about other doctors who are not directly concerned with their healthcare having access to their records. However, they are not aware of the extent to which other health staff have access to their records in their everyday work.

You may need to consider explicit negotiations with each patient to establish what information they are willing to have included in their medical records.

A young man consults you with worries about infection. He has recently discovered that the girl he had been having sex with had slept with a soldier on leave who was rumoured to have given an infection to several other girls. After discussion you arrange for him to attend the genito-urinary medicine (GUM) clinic for screening. He asks specifically that the reason for his consultation is not recorded in his medical record so, with his agreement, you enter 'health advice' as a non-specific but accurate record of his attendance.

Disclosure in the patient's own interest

You may need to give information about a patient to a relative, carer or another health professional. Normally the consent of the patient should be obtained. Occasionally, however, the clinical condition of the patient may prevent informed consent being obtained (e.g. unconsciousness, an emergency situation or severe illness).

A 16-year-old attends the family planning clinic for a pregnancy test, having had one very light period five weeks ago. The test is positive, but she is complaining of bad stomach pains. Suspecting an ectopic pregnancy, you

continued

arrange to admit her to hospital, but before you can transfer her, she collapses, appearing pale and shocked. Her friend who came with her wants you to ring her mother, but the patient has requested that no post is sent to her home, and she is not in a fit state to discuss the matter with you. If you cannot obtain consent at that time, the wishes of the patient, not those of her friend, remain your priority.

Exceptionally there may be special circumstances in which a patient should not be given medical information which could be harmful for him or her, and in such cases the information is given to a relative or carer in the best interests of the patient.

It is important to recognise that relatives or carers do *not* have any right to information about the patient. Do not breach confidentiality by giving information without consent (e.g. do not confirm a patient's attendance for treatment or give any results of investigations to someone who states that they are a relative or carer of the patient).

A social worker rings the clinic to obtain the results of vaginal swabs taken from a girl who is in the care of the local authority. She says that the girl will not attend herself and has asked for the results to be obtained, as she knows that she will have to go to the doctor if she needs treatment. Ask if you can speak to the girl herself, and explain that you cannot give information to someone else unless it is recorded that the girl has given her consent to this action.

Reassure young people about their right to confidential medical treatment. If they attend with another person, try to see them on their own at some stage. Ask them if they are happy to continue the consultation with the other person present. This can sometimes be difficult if they are accompanied by a parent or social worker. The accompanying person may be anxious that their own views are taken into consideration or even imposed. Special provision may need to be made to see parents or social workers separately, with the proviso that it is the patient's needs which are paramount.

> It is often possible to say to the person accompanying the patient 'Is there anything else you would like to ask before I see Amanda on her own?' or 'Perhaps you would like to come back in to join us after I have seen Amanda on her own?'

Including information about confidentiality in leaflets, and displaying notices about confidentiality, helps to inform people about the standards you set. Make sure that *all* staff understand the need for confidentiality, and each time anyone asks for information about others, explain the rules under which it is given. Many people have not thought about the implications of asking for someone else's results or asking if they have been seen at the surgery or clinic.

Verbal and written reports for teamworking

Increasingly, we care for patients as one member of a team. Communication with other members of that team is essential.

Disclosure required by law

Confidential information may be required by law without the consent of the patient if an Act of Parliament states that it must be disclosed in specific circumstances or for some specific purpose. For example:

> Dr N rang his defence organisation in some anxiety. He had just been served a court order to attend court with Miss M's medical record. He had read through the records and he had referred her for a termination of pregnancy four years ago. He had also written detailed notes about her account of sexual and physical abuse received from her father. The court case concerned the abuse and the father's solicitor wanted the record to show that the girl was sexually active elsewhere: in fact, the notes confirmed the girl's story. Dr N was concerned that he did not have Miss M's consent to divulge what she had told him or that she had had a termination of pregnancy. He was advised that the court order required him to break the confidence.

A Court Order may also order disclosure in a particular case. Failure to disclose information may then be illegal, although the health professional can still decline to supply information on ethical grounds and risk the legal consequences (e.g. a fine or imprisonment). If the legal requirements conflict with your ethical standpoint, seek advice from professional organisations and your professional indemnity company.

Overriding duty to society

Occasionally you may feel that your moral duty as a citizen requires you to divulge confidential information. Whenever possible you should seek to persuade the patient to give consent to the disclosure. Seek advice from professional organisations in circumstances where others are in danger (e.g. at risk of harm such as rape or sexual abuse) or where a serious crime has been committed.

An adolescent gives you information to the effect that her stepfather abused her sexually in her early teens but she never told anyone about it at the time. She is worried because he has applied to foster children. She now lives with her boyfriend's parents but is worried that he will find her and cause trouble. She does not want you to tell anyone else about her fears because she thinks it was her fault that it happened. Encourage her to express her fears of the risks to other children and realise that social services should be involved. You may be able to persuade her that Social Services must be told, but if not you must seek advice and be prepared to break her confidence in order to protect other children.

National security

Health professionals should satisfy themselves that sufficient authority has been obtained (e.g. a certificate from the Attorney General or Lord Advocate), and should consult professional organisations before disclosing information without a patient's consent.

Public health

Legislation requires notification of certain diseases and conditions to the appropriate authorities. It may sometimes be necessary, in the public interest, to disclose information in order to prevent serious risks to other people's health (e.g. communicable diseases, adverse drug reactions). Fortunately, it is only very rarely that people with sexually transmitted illnesses do not want to inform their sexual contacts or are unable to agree to a health advisor informing their contacts anonymously.

You should satisfy yourself that information is passed to someone who has a similar respect for confidentiality (not the media!).

Research

Research may benefit existing or future patients or lead to improvements in public health. Normally, confidential information about identified patients should not be used without their informed consent.

The Caldicott Committee Report[7] described the following principles of good practice for safeguarding confidentiality when information is being used for non-clinical purposes:

- justify the purpose
- do not use patient-identifiable information unless this is absolutely necessary
- always use the minimum necessary patient-identifiable information
- access to patient-identifiable information should only be available on a strict need-to-know basis
- everyone with access to patient-identifiable information should be aware of his or her responsibilities.

You should tell the subjects you invite to participate in any consultation or survey about the standards of confidentiality, and you should inform them about the extent to which their identity, contact details and the information which they give you is confidential to you, your work team or your organisation.

If you are running a focus group or other small-group work, you should suggest a code of practice to the group, and then seek their agreement or ask the group to formulate their own modification. The rules should include agreement about confidentiality and exactly what information may or may not be repeated outside the group. Establish precisely what information may be freely repeated so long as it is not attributed to named individuals.

If researchers who require information about patients approach you for data from your patients' records, you should not disclose it unless informed consent has been given or that consent is not required after consideration by an appropriate ethical committee. You should not disclose information if you are aware that the patient would withhold their consent if they were asked for it.

Teaching

The patient's informed consent should be obtained before sharing any personal information required for teaching. Students should be made aware of the importance of confidentiality and its preservation. Video-recording is frequently used for teaching and learning. Explain clearly to patients the purpose, use and audience with regard to such recordings, and give them an unpressurised opportunity to decline or to request erasure of the recording.

Family planning clinics often have doctors or nurses in training. Patients should always have the option to be seen without the trainee present, and should not be made to feel that they are being pressurised into agreeing.

Is a notice on the wall by reception stating that this is a teaching clinic or practice sufficient? You might introduce a card on which patients can tick 'yes' or 'no' in answer to the question 'Do you object to a doctor or nurse in training being present when you are seen?'. The card is handed back to the receptionist, who then notifies the health professional of the patient's wishes.

Management responsibility

A written confidentiality policy document should be drawn to the attention of *all* staff including any staff at induction or in training. They should understand and preferably sign the confidentiality policy statement. Access to it should be encouraged and appropriate training provided.[5]

A named person should be responsible for updating the policy document, monitoring adherence to it, and dealing with any potential or actual breaches of confidentiality.

Temporary, voluntary or work-experience students should all be informed of their obligations to maintain confidentiality; they should be given a copy of a simplified policy stating their obligations to preserve confidentiality. Interpreters should be used wherever possible to avoid the use of friends or relatives in this capacity, and they should be trained in the requirements of confidentiality.

Managers must ensure that paper and computer security is maintained and systems for monitoring and upgrading security systems put into practice.

Management, clerical and administrative staff responsibilities for confidentiality include the following:

- a clause about confidentiality in contracts of employment
- training in issues of confidentiality for all staff
- a named person with whom any member of staff can discuss difficulties with regard to confidentiality, such as emotional pressure, financial inducement or lapses (their own or those of others)
- reporting physical difficulties such as lack of privacy at reception desks or being overheard answering the telephone
- having clear rules about the handling of post marked 'private', 'confidential' or 'personal'
- explaining the reasons for requests for information from patients, and only seeking the minimum amount of information required for the task
- shredding of confidential paper records.

Secure storage of records

The policy document on confidentiality should describe clear procedures for recording and storing information on paper and/or on computer. Safeguards against unauthorised access to either form of data must be built in and tested. Personal medical data must be stored separately from financial, administrative and research data.[8]

Levels of access to data should be clearly stated and passwords to computer records kept confidential (and not left on a sticky label on the computer terminal!). Terminal security must be arranged so that no unattended terminal can be used by an unauthorised person to access data.

Modem security must provide 'firewall' security against unauthorised access to confidential data. Information technology makes sensitive data readily available – not just to those who need to access it.

Transmission of records and information

Consider the security of fax[9] or electronic data before using this method of transmission. Do you know who will see the information at the other end?

If information is requested by telephone, do you know the identity of the person to whom you are speaking? Are you absolutely sure it is not a journalist pretending to be a medical secretary?

Think about conflicts

- Medical information is confidential – yet employers and social security officers expect a signed diagnosis if someone is absent from work.

> A 15-year-old is supposed to have work experience the week that she is due to be admitted for a termination of pregnancy. She wants a note to explain why she has to
>
> *continued*

be absent, but does not want the termination to be mentioned. You might use a euphemism such as 'hospital treatment'.

- Medical information is confidential – yet relatives expect to be informed if someone is terminally ill or suffering from a serious illness.

A 16-year-old attends for emergency contraception and decides on an intra-uterine device. During the fitting, she collapses and has to be admitted to hospital. She lives at home, but does not want her parents to be told because they disapprove of her boyfriend. She needs to be aware of the implications and difficulties inherent in concealing what has happened. After discussion, you should offer to support whatever decision she finally makes.

- Medical information is confidential – yet patients expect a full and informative letter to be sent with any request for a specialist opinion, but have reservations about secretaries or receptionists seeing their medical records.

An 18-year-old complains because she was given her appointment and referral letter to the hospital for a termination of pregnancy by the clerk at the clinic. She knows that the clerk has a sister who works in the same hairdressing salon as she does, and she feels that confidentiality has been compromised. You should explain that the clerk is bound by the same rules of confidentiality as yourself, and would lose her job if those rules were breached.

- Medical information is confidential – yet patients give signed consent for their doctors to give full details from their medical records to insurance companies, but at the same time expect their doctors to withhold any information that would have adverse consequences.[10]

> A 19-year-old is taking out a mortgage with her husband. She has asked to see the medical report before it goes to the insurance company, because she has had problems with a whiplash injury. She is horrified to discover that the referral by a previous general practitioner to the GUM clinic three years previously and her termination of pregnancy the following year are both recorded, and asks for them to be deleted from her report. She needs to be aware that you have to sign the form stating whether or not the information it contains has been modified at her request. She may need to be offered some help with sorting out her feelings about these events if she is so horrified that others may find out about them.

If health workers are confused, it is no wonder that patients are!

Further reading

BMA Handbook Working Party (1988) *Philosophy and Practice of Medical Ethics*. British Medical Association, London.

Egg Research and Consultancy (1999) *You think they won't tell anyone, well you HOPE they won't ... Do young people believe sex advice is CONFIDENTIAL?* Brook Advisory Centres/Royal College of General Practitioners, London.

Woodrow P (1996) Exploring confidentiality in nursing practice. *Nursing Standard*. **10**: 38–42.

References

1   Donovan C, Mellanby AR, Jacobson LD, Taylor B and Tripp JH (1997) Teenagers' views on the general practice consultation and provision of contraception. *Br J Gen Pract*. **47**: 715–18.

2 Ford CA, Millstein SG, Halpern-Felsher BL and Irwin CE (1997) Influence of physician confidentiality assurances on adolescents' willingness to disclose information and seek future healthcare. *JAMA*. **278**: 1029–34.

3 Hutchinson F (1993) Contraceptive needs of young people. *Br J Sex Med*. **20**: 10–12.

4 Jacobson L (2000) Teenagers do not trust GPs on confidential consultations. *Pulse (news)*. **29 April**: 12.

5 Royal College of General Practitioners/Brook Advisory Centres (2000) *Confidentiality and Young People. Improving Teenagers' Uptake of Health Advice: a toolkit for general practices and primary care groups/trusts*. RCGP/Brook Advisory Centres in conjunction with the RCN, BMA, GPC, DoH, MDU, London.

6 Department of Health (2000) *Contraceptive Services for Under 16-year-olds: new guidance for health professionals*. Health Service Circular (in press). Department of Health, London.

7 Department of Health (1997) Report of the review of patient-identifiable information. In: *The Caldicott Committee Report*. Department of Health, London.

8 Fisher F and Madge B (1996) Data security and patient confidentiality. *Int J Biomed Computing*. **43**: 115–19.

9 Genesen L *et al.* (1994) Faxing medical records: another threat to confidentiality in medicine. *JAMA*. **271**: 1401–2.

10 Lorge RE (1989) How informed is patient's consent to the release of medical information to insurance companies? *BMJ*. **298**: 1495–96.

► CHAPTER 6

Contraception for teenagers

Special considerations when seeing young people[1]

- Discuss the guidelines on confidentiality with all young people.
- Always offer the young person the option of being seen alone.
- Follow up young people more frequently initially in order to build trust and confidence.
- Only consider a pelvic examination if pathology is suspected.
- Know the local procedure for Child Protection in case you find out that a young person is at risk of suffering or significant harm (*also see* Chapter 13 on abuse).
- Know and follow the 'Gillick or Fraser rules' for advice and prescription for those under 16-years-old[2], and the recent HSC[3] (*also see* Chapter 5 on confidentiality where the rules are described in detail).

Be proactive. If you do not know what method of contraception a young person is using, then ask!

The new clearer guidance for all health professionals[3] includes a framework for the counselling that should accompany the prescription, supply or administration of contraceptives to a person under 16 without the knowledge of their parent or carer. This should cover:

- the case for a discussion with a parent or carer
- relationship with partner including possible coercion or abuse (to include the age of the partner and discussion of the law)

- the arguments for delaying sexual activity
- sources of counselling, help and support on issues raised.

Contraceptive consultations

Unless individuals wish to use a particular method, they will abandon it later. It is therefore important to:

- explore the patient's ideas about contraception as well as those of their partner
- use a checklist to select out those patients for whom a particular method would not be safe (*see* Table 6.1) or consult the more detailed summary list in the Royal College of General Practitioners' *Handbook of Sexual Health in Primary Care*[4]
- negotiate an acceptable method
- teach the method using visual aids such as leaflets and models, and check understanding
- arrange how to obtain supplies, when to return routinely, and the safety-net to be used if things do not go according to plan, e.g. missed pills
- use any spare time for health promotion (advice on safe sex, smoking, diet and exercise, etc.), but remember that the prime concern is the provision of contraception.

Choice of method

No one method will suit everyone, and individuals will choose different methods at different stages of their lives. No ideal method exists, and all methods can fail – some more often than others. If it is important to avoid pregnancy, then a more reliable method should be chosen. Keep a good up-to-date reference manual handy, such as the fpa's (previously known as the Family Planning Association) *Contraceptive Handbook*,[5] or other authoritative text[6] to consult if any problems or queries arise.

It is important to discuss some of the less reliable but neglected methods. It is assumed that young people will want to use the combined oral contraceptive pill and condoms or the

Table 6.1: Checklist – if these conditions are present either the method should not be used [X] or you should check a reference book or the data sheet for relative contraindications or cautions [C]

	Method of contraception*						
Medical condition	COC	POP	Injection	Implant	IUD	IUS	Barrier
Pregnancy	X	X	X	X	X	X	
Before any pregnancies					C	C	
Hypertension	X						
Structural heart disease with significant valve problem or a septal defect	X				C		
Bacterial endocarditis (past or at risk)					X	X	
Known high risk of thrombosis due to inherited condition or immobility	X						
Inherited hyperlipidaemia	X/C						
Migraine with focal symptoms	X						
Irregular vaginal bleeding before diagnosis of cause	X	X	X	X	X	X	
Heavy or painful menstrual loss					C		
Ovarian cyst		C					
Previous ectopic pregnancy		C			C		
Septate uterus or stenosis of cervical os					X	X	
Pelvic inflammatory disease or increased risk					X	X	
Toxic shock syndrome							C
Recurrent urinary tract infections							C
Biliary tract disease or cholestasis	C	C	C	C		C	
Liver disease current or before tests have returned to normal	X	C	C	C		C	
Porphyria	X						
Wilson's disease					X		
Liver tumours	X	C	C	C		C	
Thalassaemia					C		
Sickle-cell disease (not sickle-cell *trait*, which can be disregarded)	C				C		
Anaemias					C		
Drug interactions (with rifampicin, phenytoin, carbamazepine, barbiturates, topiramate, ritonavir or other liver-enzyme inducers)	C	C	C	C			

* COC: combined oral contraceptive; IUD: intrauterine device; Injection: progestogen injectable method; Barrier: diaphragm, cap, condoms; POP: progestogen-only pill; IUS: intra-uterine system with progestogen; Implant: progestogen implant.

injection, because these are the methods that health professionals would like them to use for maximum contraceptive efficacy. Sexual activity is enjoyable, but contraception is a nuisance and will be neglected or avoided unless it is the choice made by the individual concerned. Knowing that all possibilities have been considered, the teenager is not left thinking 'There must be something better than this' or 'I'm not having sex often, so I won't bother with all this stuff'.

Abstinence

The effectiveness of this method is 100% if it is used reliably, and 10–20% per episode if not (i.e. the background risk of becoming pregnant if no contraceptive method is used, and the couple do not abstain after all).[7]

Abstinence means choosing not to have sexual intercourse at all (not just sometimes!). This is very difficult when passions are running high in the teenage years, and it requires a co-operative partner who is in agreement with the method. Abstinence from sexual penetration only works if both partners trust the other to abide by the rules. If one person cannot trust the other, then complete avoidance of sexual touching is necessary. Abstinence may range from no body contact at all to holding hands, kissing and petting or even having oral sex. The important point is that there is no contact at all between the penis and the female genital area. The male partner produces ejaculate containing sperm (and sometimes other undesirable things like infection) long before ejaculation. Advising young people about this method should involve discussion of issues such as what other forms of sexual release that couple might want (e.g. masturbation), and being able to discuss other forms of sexual expression that do not involve genital contact.

Abstinence is particularly suitable for people who are still undecided about a sexual relationship, who have religious beliefs about chastity or when both partners agree. It is not ideal, but is possible when periodic abstinence is combined with so-called 'natural' fertility control methods. The couple should proceed with caution if agreement is obtained in principle but found to be very difficult to adhere to, and the method is contra-indicated if agreement between the couple is not forthcoming.

> M had been brought up in the Sikh religion. She became very fond of another student at college, who was of a different faith. They both knew that they could not marry and that according to her religion she should remain a virgin until her marriage. M attended a clinic in a different town to her own, very fearfully, seeking emergency contraception after the couple had not been able to control themselves sufficiently.

A study showed that compared to the usual sex education programmes, abstinence programmes in schools did not have any additional effect in delaying sexual activity or reducing pregnancy.[1] Abstinence cannot be imposed on people against their will!

Periodic abstinence or 'natural fertility control methods'

Failure rates are difficult to establish because of the varying levels of application of these methods, but are usually quoted to be between about 2% and 20% per annum.[7] In addition, there is absolutely no protection against STDs.

A number of indicators can be used. The more indicators that are used, the more reliable is the method. It depends on *predicting ovulation* (which usually occurs about 12–16 days *before* the next menstrual period in a regular cycle). Cycle length alone (the calendar method) is the least reliable way of predicting ovulation, but can be combined with:

- waking body temperature
- cervical secretions (mucus)
- fertility devices that measure hormone changes (e.g. Persona).

All of these methods need to be accurately taught over several cycles for best practice, and they depend on the couple abstaining during the fertile days, or using barrier methods intermittently.

Teenagers often ask about this method and have inadequate information about its effectiveness or otherwise. After full counselling, they often decide that it is not a method that they can rely upon. Using a fertility predictor such as Persona is also rather expensive for the average teenager, as this device is not available on the NHS. Restriction of intercourse to the time after ovulation has occurred makes it a much more reliable method, but is unlikely to be successful in any but the most self-controlled and obsessive adolescent couple!

The other 'natural method' that is often neglected is *fully* breastfeeding (using no supplements and feeding on demand day and night) up to six months after delivery and before menstruation has returned. This is only suitable for baby-spacing in older teenagers who are in stable, well-supported relationships, but it is better than nothing for an unsupported teenage mother embarking on a new relationship! In reality few teenage mothers manage *full* breastfeeding without using some supplements.

Withdrawal (coitus interruptus)

It is difficult to establish the reliability of this method. Studies have mainly been conducted on couples in stable long-term relationships, in whom the fertility rate does not seem to be increased compared to groups using barrier methods.

Withdrawal is a commonly used method and is better than no contraception at all in an emergency. It should perhaps be more widely discussed, as many people who are just starting to become sexually active have given no thought to contraception until after penetration. This method would certainly have an impact on teenage pregnancy rates if it was regarded as something in which young men should become expert!

The main disadvantage of this method is the control necessary to withdraw before ejaculation. For many couples this appears to have no adverse psychological effects, but others complain that it leaves them feeling incomplete or frustrated. The need to predict the moment of orgasm may be particularly problematic for young men, who often experience premature ejaculation and have yet to learn control over the mechanisms for delaying ejaculation. Some sperm may be present in the pre-ejaculate fluid, which can contribute to the perceived high failure rate.

There are many other more reliable methods, but this one is (sometimes) possible in an emergency! It should preferably be backed up by rapid access to emergency contraceptive methods (within 24 hours if possible), and consideration of more long-term methods.

Combined oral contraceptive (COC) pills

With regard to the failure rate, many figures have been quoted, ranging from 0.1% to 5% per annum.[7] The fpa quotes a figure of 99% contraceptive safety with consistent use.

The low failure rate, lack of interference with sexual activity and regular lighter periods associated with its use make this an attractive method. Improvement of teenage acne with oestrogen-dominant pills is an important selling point! Record the history you take in order to exclude those patients who are unsuitable for hormonal contraception, and update it regularly. Most young women will have no contraindications to the use of COCs, and after taking a history and checking their blood pressure you can concentrate on ensuring that they know how to use it. Do not assume that they will know – many people misunderstand, or remember incorrectly, information that was acquired when it was not so important.

Young people are generally uninterested in the long-term effects of COCs, but you should always ask if they have any worries and, if so, discuss them in detail in order to prevent early discontinuation. It is often more time-efficient to postpone detailed discussion of cardiovascular risks, breast cancer and smoking until later visits, when these can be assimilated and weighed against the benefits of COCs. Use the first consultation to convey essential information about how to take the pill and how to cope with minor side-effects. Finding out what the teenager already knows, or thinks she knows, about the pill helps you to focus your information on any misunderstandings or incorrect knowledge.

Information about missed pills needs frequent repetition, backed up by a leaflet. Emphasise the risks of lengthening the pill-free week to more than seven days. By the end of the pill-free week, follicles may only be a couple of days away from being ripe enough to release the ovum, and they only become quiescent on restarting the COC. Fortunately, this degree of activity only occurs in a few women, but nearly 25% of women show some ovarian follicular activity by the seventh pill-free day. Using a chart (*see* Figure 6.1) to illustrate the risks can help to clarify them.

Discuss where the young woman will keep her pills if she is living at home. If she has to conceal them from other family members (especially younger brothers) she may be more likely to forget them. Building in reminder mechanisms (e.g. keeping the packet with her clean underwear or her toothbrush)

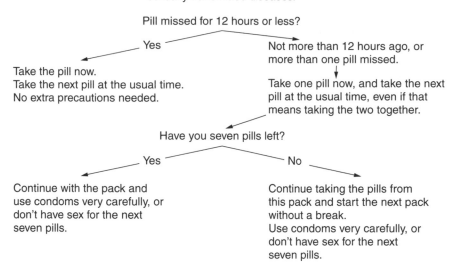

If you have always used condoms, you have added safety against pregnancy and sexually transmitted diseases.

Pill missed for 12 hours or less?

Yes

Not more than 12 hours ago, or more than one pill missed.

Take the pill now.
Take the next pill at the usual time.
No extra precautions needed.

Take one pill now, and take the next pill at the usual time, even if that means taking the two together.

Have you seven pills left?

Yes

No

Continue with the pack and use condoms very carefully, or don't have sex for the next seven pills.

Continue taking the pills from this pack and start the next pack without a break.
Use condoms very carefully, or don't have sex for the next seven pills.

If you start taking antibiotics you may not absorb as much of the pill as usual, so use condoms very carefully while you are taking the antibiotics and for seven days afterwards.

If you are taking long-term antibiotics for acne, the effects on absorption of the pill will wear off after the first two weeks, so you will not need to continue with extra precautions against pregnancy, only against sexually transmitted diseases.

Figure 6.1: Missed pill rules.

may aid regular pill-taking. Enlist the help of her best friend, as most teenagers see their best friend more often than their boyfriend, and they often come to the consultation together. Some pills are produced in an everyday package with dummy pills for the seven pill-free days. These have not been particularly popular in the UK, mainly because of the risks associated with missed pills around that hormone-free week and the complicated instructions that are needed if pills are forgotten or vomited.

COCs are particularly suitable for healthy young women with good memories and organised lives. They are not ideal but represent a possible option for those with chaotic lifestyles or anxiety about the method. You should consult a reliable check-list as recommended above for relative or absolute medical contraindications.

Progestogen-only contraceptive pills (POPs)

The failure rate of this method is about 2–3% per annum with consistent use.[7]

The need to take POPs at a regular time makes them less attractive for the young or for those with chaotic lifestyles. However, do not underestimate a woman's ability to take the POPs consistently if she chooses to use this method. POPs have to be taken at the same time every day without a break, and this sometimes makes them easier to remember than a pill with a one-week break. The current fashion for not carrying a handbag and for clothing with tight pockets may make carrying the pills difficult, so you should discuss daily access to the place where the pills are kept.

> D keeps her pills at her best friend's house and keeps just a spare packet in her own drawer at home. She shares her bedroom at home with two younger sisters, so she often spends the night with her best friend, who has the luxury of a room to herself with two beds.

POPs are particularly suitable for the few women for whom COCs pose health risks. Although women with diabetes can take COCs, they usually have a regular lifestyle that is well suited to taking POPs. Patients with mobility problems, such as those confined to wheelchairs, can safely avoid the increased thrombosis risk associated with oestrogen by using POPs.

However, it is important to be cautious about the use of POPs in obese women (BMI > 30) who have an increased thrombosis risk with oestrogen. Body weight over 70 kg appears to be associated with a higher failure rate, and you may need to consider prescribing two pills daily (although this is an unlicensed treatment).

POPs are particularly suitable for women with good memories and regular lifestyles, and for those with contra-indications to oestrogen. They are not ideal but are a possible method for those with irregular lifestyles or who are obese. If there are health problems, consult Table 6.1 or an authoritative text.[6,7] Bear in mind that many of the exclusions for POPs have been drawn from extrapolation of evidence about COCs, and that you may need to seek expert advice in difficult clinical situations.

Injectable progestogens

The failure rate for this method is less than 1% per annum.[7]

Depo-Provera (medroxyprogesterone acetate) and Noristerat (norethisterone oenathate) are extremely effective contraceptives when given punctually every 12 weeks. Injections are particularly suitable for women who have heavy periods, for those who find it difficult to remember to take pills or after failure of other methods. Injections are also a useful method for those who would have difficulty storing medication (e.g. people who are homeless, living in hostels or sharing a room with others). Women with learning difficulties or with disabilities, who may have problems managing hygiene during their periods, may welcome the amenorrhoea or light loss that usually occurs.

W is now living in a hostel after leaving a children's home when she was 16-years-old. She has a very 'on-off' relationship with a boy who lives in another town who she rarely sees. Despite this, she prefers to have regular Depo-Provera injections so that 'nobody knows her business'. She finds the lack of periods much easier to manage in the communal environment of the hostel. Her ambition is to have a room of her own where she can shut the door on the world and be in control of her own space.

It is important to provide counselling about the usually infrequent or absent periods and the management of early irregular bleeding (*see* Table 6.2), in order to achieve good continuation rates. You must ensure that the woman has had ample opportunity to discuss any fears or queries about the method before giving an injection, as the treatment cannot be discontinued by the user within the next three months if she has second thoughts!

Arrange how to set up reminder mechanisms for those few patients who are really unreliable about remembering to return after 12 weeks. Consider reducing the interval between injections if the patient often attends late, and ensure that you know how to manage late attendance (*see* Table 6.3).

Table 6.2: Management of bleeding problems

1 Clarify the extent of bleeding
2 If within 4–8 weeks of the last injection, consider adding the combined pill (COC) for 21 days*
3 If 8 or more weeks have elapsed since last injection, consider repeat injection*
4 Consider other causes (chlamydia, cervical ectopy, etc.)
5 Consider alternative methods of contraception if this method is unacceptable

* Evidence for these routines is lacking, but they are commonly followed.

Table 6.3: Management of late attendance for Depo-Provera injection

	Time elapsed since last injection			
	Up to 12 weeks + 5 days (i.e. 89 days)	89–94 days	Up to 14 weeks (i.e. 94–98 days)	After 14 weeks (i.e. 98+ days)
If patient has had unprotected sexual intercourse	Not at risk	Give post-coital oral contraception	Fit post-coital IUD	Assume patient is at risk of pregnancy
Barrier methods	Always advise use if injection is delayed for any reason			
Pregnancy test	No	Yes	Yes	Yes, and repeat in two weeks
Give injection	Yes	Yes, if test is negative	Yes, if test is negative	Only after a second negative test

Progestogen implants

The failure rate for this method is very low. It is probably as reliable a method as sterilisation (but it is still relatively new, so we await more widespread use for definitive results).

Norplant has now been discontinued by the manufacturers. The need for surgical insertion of six rods and their visibility in the skin of the upper arm deterred some women from using it, whilst others wore it like a badge proclaiming their protection. The rods need to be removed after five years of use by a doctor trained in the removal technique.

Implanon has recently been introduced. It has only one rod about the size of a hairgrip, so both insertion and removal are easier. It can be felt under the skin, but is less visible than Norplant as it lies in the groove between the muscles. It is inserted just under the skin on the upper arm with a special introducer under local anaesthetic. It can remain in place for three years and then be removed under local anaesthetic by making a small cut in the skin and pulling out the plastic carrier rod.

Adequate counselling about progestogenic side-effects, especially the irregular bleeding, reduces removal rates. Blood levels are similar to those with the progestogen-only pills, and the side-effects are about the same, but without the need for a good memory!

A progestogen implant is particularly suitable for women who want a long-term, reliable method. It may be less acceptable if irregular periods are undesirable for any reason or if the patient is afraid of minor surgical procedures. Contra-indications are the same as for any progestogen-only method.

Intrauterine devices (IUDs)

The failure rate for this method is less than 1% in the first year.[7]

The risk of chlamydial infection and pelvic infection is increased in the young and in those who have had more than two partners in the last 12 months.[8] Consider taking high vaginal swabs (with informed consent) before fitting an IUD, especially in higher-risk patients (*see* Chapter 10 on sexual diseases and allied problems). The risk of infection associated with an IUD is mainly due to the fitting, when bacteria from the vagina may be conveyed to the uterus. A sexual history and an estimate of the risk of changes of partner must be balanced against the effectiveness of the method.

The choice of IUDs in general practice may be limited by which ones are on the drug tariff. Devices that have less than $300\,mm^2$ surface area of copper are associated with a higher pregnancy rate than those with a larger surface area of copper.

The Copper T380 series is associated with low pregnancy rates, with the Multiload 375 coming a close second. Both of these devices are easier to fit after a full-term delivery. Gynaefix (a frameless device consisting of copper tubes fixed into the fundus of the uterus with a knot) requires special training to fit, and the Nova T380Ag that replaces the Nova T (200) is not yet on the drug tariff to be prescribed.

Nova T or the Multiload 250 are only suitable for short-term use, but the Nova T has a narrow inserter and is much easier to insert for post-coital use in women who have had no babies.

IUDs are more suitable for stable long-term relationships, for spacing pregnancies, and for long-term use after the family is complete. But don't deny teenagers the opportunity of selecting IUDs as their method of choice if they understand the relative risks.

Emergency contraception

Make sure that *all* staff and patients know how to obtain emergency contraception and the time limits involved. You can increase the availability of emergency contraception by using protocols so that suitably trained nurses can see patients if a doctor is unavailable. Table 6.4 lists some guidelines[9] that can be used as a basis for protocol production.

The two hormonal methods, PC4 and Levonelle-2, can be used up to 72 hours after unprotected intercourse, but the earlier the better. PC4 contains both oestrogen and progestogen and is associated with a higher rate of nausea and vomiting than Levonelle-2, which only contains progestogen.

In trials comparing the two methods,[10] the progestogen-only method had a lower failure rate than the combined pill, especially when taken within 24 hours of exposure as described in Table 6.5 on p. 94.

Don't forget that larger doses of hormone (probably three pills of PC4 twice or two pills of Levonelle-2 twice) are necessary for patients on hepatic enzyme inducers such as phenytoin, carbamazepine or rifampicin in order to obtain the same blood levels.

Legislation is now in place in England to allow pharmacists to supply emergency contraceptive pills[11] without the woman having been seen by a doctor first. This is likely to encourage local schemes to fund pharmacists to supply free emergency contraceptives as pharmacy medicines.

The insertion of a copper IUD up to 5 days after unprotected intercourse has an even lower failure rate (0.1%).

Table 6.4: Emergency contraception: basis for a protocol

Minimum information to be recorded in the notes prior to prescribing oral post-coital contraception should include the following:
- last menstrual period (LMP)
- cycle length
- date and time of unprotected sexual intercourse (UPSI)
- day of cycle of UPSI
- any other UPSI since LMP
- options discussed (oral/IUD)
- any interacting medication
- current liver disease
- history of thromboembolism
- focal migraine at the time when PCC is required.

Counselling should include the following:
- likelihood of nausea
- mode of action
- failure rate
- side-effects
- timing of next period
- action to take if next period is not on time
- discussion of future contraception needs.

Vomiting after taking emergency combined oral contraception
If the patient vomits within two hours of taking the pills, she should be advised to seek further medical advice. Domperidone, 10 mg, can be used to prevent vomiting.

Issuing guidelines
- Negotiate the times of the first and second doses and write them down.
- Go through the leaflet with the patient.
- Make follow-up arrangements or advise the patient to return one week after the expected date of the next period.
- Give or prescribe emergency contraception.

It can be used up to 5 days after the calculated date of ovulation (i.e. the nineteenth day of a 28-day shortest cycle by history, counting day 1 as the first day of bleeding) and it successfully prevents implantation. Remember that exposure to unprotected intercourse also involves exposure to possible infection, so informed consent for screening, especially for chlamydial infection, is usually required. The IUD can be removed at the

Table 6.5: Effectiveness of two different types of oral emergency contraception

Time interval between coitus and treatment	Percentage of expected pregnancies prevented by emergency contraception	
	Combined oestrogen/ progestogen (%)	Progestogen only (%)
24 hours or less	77	95
25–48 hours	36	85
49–72 hours	31	58

next menstruation if it is neither required nor desired for continuing contraception.

Condoms

The failure rates for this method are 3% for perfect use and 14% for typical typical use per annum.[6]

Not all general practices are able to provide condoms as family planning clinics are, but it is important to be aware of the types that are available. Different sizes and shapes suit different sizes and shapes of men. If they are unable to supply them, health professionals should know where condoms can be obtained free of charge to the user (e.g. family planning clinics). This method should also be recommended for those who are likely to change partners. Discuss with the patient how they can negotiate the use of condoms with their partner, and how to obtain emergency contraception in the event of a failure.

Health professionals and other providers of condoms need to be comfortable discussing how a condom should be used and suggesting ways in which it can be incorporated into love play. Advice should be given on the use of water-based lubricants (not lubricants containing oil, which can weaken the latex), which can reduce tearing and irritation as well as increasing sensitivity. An even better option is to use a spermicide-containing lubricant which may further reduce the risk if spillage or tearing does occur. (Don't believe the myth that condoms burst – the average condom stretches to about 150 centimetres (5 feet) in length and can hold 16 pints of beer!) Instruction should include how to hold the base of the condom after climax and before withdrawing to prevent spillage, and how to dispose of used condoms!

> R wanted to know whether it was safe to use condoms after having a massage, as his girlfriend was learning aromatherapy. He was advised that massage oils could weaken the condom if it was exposed to them for any length of time. It was suggested that the couple might like to have a shower or bath together before having intercourse, to continue the relaxation and closeness that he enjoyed.

Female condoms (Femidom) need to be used carefully to avoid positioning the penis so that it is not covered. They are rather expensive, but can be bought over the counter with no need for medical intervention. They are disliked by some because of their 'plastic mac' feel and the fact that they are noisy in use; but others opt for them as a barrier method under the woman's control.

Diaphragms and caps

The failure rates are 5% for perfect use and 21% for typical use per annum.[6]

Fitting a diaphragm involves having a vaginal examination, and this may deter some women. The diaphragm must always be used together with a spermicide. Good teaching and practice are essential to ensure that the diaphragm and pool of spermicide cover the cervix.

The degree of organisation and forward planning required for reliable use of this method makes the diaphragm a more suitable choice for individuals in stable long-term relationships. It also requires access to (preferably private) washing facilities and a convenient place for storage.

References

1   Cooper P, Diamond I, High S and Pearson S (1994) A comparison of family planning provision: general practice and family planning clinics. *Br J Fam Plan*. **19**: 263–9.

2   Family Planning Association (1993) Guidance issued jointly on confidentiality and people under 16. British Medical Association, GMSC, Health Education Authority, Brook Advisory Centres, Family Planning Association and Royal College of General Practitioners, London.

3   Department of Health (2000) *Contraceptive Services for Under 16-year-olds: new guidance for health professionals*. Health Service Circular (in press). Department of Health, London.

4   Carter Y, Moss C and Weyman A (eds) (1998) *Handbook of Sexual Health in Primary Care*. Royal College of General Practitioners, London.

5   Belfield T (1999) *Contraceptive Handbook* (3e). Family Planning Association, London.

6   Guillebaud J (1999) *Contraception: Your Questions Answered* (3e). Churchill Livingstone, London.

7   Trussel J (1998) Contraceptive efficacy. In: J Trussel, F Stewart, W Cates *et al.* (eds) *Contraceptive Technology* (17e). Ardent Media, New York.

8   Scholes D, Stergachis A, Heindrich FE *et al.* (1996) Prevention of pelvic inflammatory disease by screening for cervical chlamydial infection. *NEJM*. **334**: 1362–6.

9   Faculty of Family Planning and Reproductive Healthcare, RCOG (2000) Emergency contraception: recommendations for clinical practice. *Br J Fam Plan*. **26**: 93–6.

10 Task Force on Postovulatory Methods of Fertility Regulation (1998) Randomised controlled trial of levonorgestrel versus the Yuzpe regimen of combined oral contraceptives for emergency contraception. *Lancet*. **352**: 428–33.

11 Department of Health (2000) *Patient Group Directions* (England only). Health Service Circular 2000/026. Department of Health, London.

CHAPTER 7

The experience of being pregnant and a parent as a young person

There are many young people who do make positive choices to conceive, for social and personal reasons. Teenage girls are encouraged to become mothers in some religions and cultures. We should aim to give such young people reliable information and easy access to effective contraception, advice and support, so that they can make informed choices about the timing of sex and pregnancy and prepare for parenthood. They need time and support to think through the implications of having a baby at a young age. Such considerations include the material possessions they will need to accumulate, how their career prospects will be affected, the limitations on their social and leisure lives, how they will sustain their relationship as a couple, and the level of household income they will need to bring up a young family and avoid poverty.

One group who positively want to be teenage parents are those living in local authority care, known as 'looked-after' young people. They are twice as likely to want to have a baby by the time they are 20-years-old as those young people who live with their families.[1]

The male partners of pregnant teenage girls tend to be older than the girls. Thus any initiatives designed to reduce teenage conception rates or support teenage pregnancies should be targeted at slightly older men, in their early twenties, otherwise the male partners may be missed by the programme. In one study, the male partner's positive attitude and indication of support was found to be a strong influence on the pregnant girl's decision to proceed with the pregnancy and attend for antenatal care or opt for a termination.[2]

Support and advice in making choices in early pregnancy

Around 75% of teenage pregnancies are unplanned.[1] A study of 113 teenage girls giving birth in one hospital over a three-month period found that one-third of them had intended to become pregnant, another third had not used contraception, and the remainder attributed their pregnancy to a failure of contraception.[3] Only one of the 57 teenage girls who had a termination at the hospital during the study period had intended to become pregnant.

A major priority in any local initiative should be to encourage young people to seek advice early if they think that they might be pregnant. The statistics for terminations performed in the UK show that disproportionately more young women have later terminations (*see* Chapter 8 on unplanned pregnancy). Counselling can help teenage girls and their partners who wish to proceed with their pregnancies – just as much as those who choose to terminate – to prepare for future parenthood, discuss and decide on future contraception, and start working out a plan to resume education and continue with a career.

In one study of 75 pregnant teenagers in the Grampian region, those teenagers who opted for termination had statistically significantly higher levels of education compared to those who presented for antenatal care.[2]

There is very haphazard availability of advice and support for helping the pregnant teenage girl and her partner to decide whether to proceed with the pregnancy, have a termination or place the baby for adoption, and in the former case, how to cope with a continuing pregnancy and start planning for a future with a child.[1] Many teenagers find it difficult to tell their parents that they are pregnant. For instance, about half of the teenagers who phone Childline for advice have told their friends but not their parents, as opposed to one in 10 teenagers who have already told their parents before phoning Childline.[1]

Sure Start schemes run by Social Services departments are targeted at helping young people to work through these issues. Sure Start is a new scheme designed to co-ordinate help for families in greatest need, through 250 local schemes established across England. An outreach worker will visit every family within three months of a baby's birth. Sure Start provides support for parents such as training for work and help with parenting problems.

Few pregnant teenagers consider giving up their babies for adoption these days. There has been a significant downward

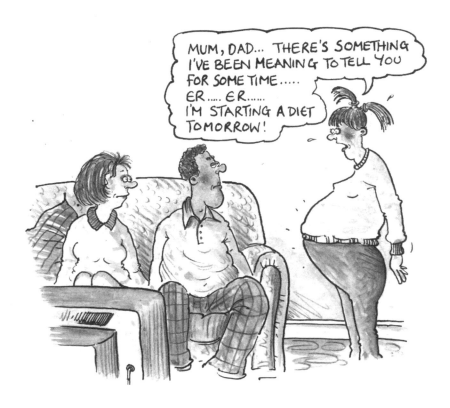

trend in the number of babies being placed for adoption at all maternal ages. In 1996, 5200 babies were adopted – a quarter of the number adopted in 1975.[1]

One study of 84 women who had their first babies when they were aged between 16 and 19 years found that the majority had not planned their pregnancies, but continued with those pregnancies because of a passive and fatalistic acceptance of the situation, rather than because they had made a positive decision.[1] Many of these teenage mothers had had unrealistic expectations both that their relationship with the baby's father would continue, and about the reality of teenage parenthood. One year on, 50% of the relationships with the babies' fathers had broken down.

Antenatal health and care

Pregnant teenagers fare less well with regard to their antenatal health than older women. This is mainly due to late presentation for the first appointment for antenatal care, and because a disproportionate number of pregnant teenagers have risk factors for poorer antenatal health (e.g. living in poverty and smoking cigarettes). One study of pregnant teenagers reported that nearly two-thirds had smoked before their pregnancy and about half continued to do so while pregnant. Fewer pregnant young women have been found to take folic acid supplements compared to those in older age groups, and young people are less likely to attend antenatal and parentcraft classes – especially young people who are being cared for by the local authority.

Limits to education and a career

Some schools do not help pregnant teenagers to continue their school education, and exclusion often means a permanent discontinuation of education. The government is now exerting more pressure on local education authorities to provide full-time education for any children who are out of school for three weeks, which should improve the educational prospects for teenage mothers in future.

The Social Exclusion Unit Report emphasises how difficult life is for young mothers and their partners who are trying to care for a child, resenting the loss of their social life and encountering innumerable barriers to gaining qualifications or being able to work. Child-care costs may be prohibitively high, and dependable child care may be non-existent. It can be a very isolated life, living away from their parents' home in a flat of their own, with the baby or child preventing the young parent(s) from socialising with their peers or being able to go out to work.

> Teenage parents get little of the right support – help back into education, into a job, proper housing, and advice on how to be a good parent – and are too often given state support that isolates them from what they need most. This makes it all the more likely that they will remain isolated and on benefit for longer than they need to be.[1]

Various 'New Deal' schemes aim to help people from deprived communities to improve their job prospects. The New Deal for Lone Parents scheme is aimed at those with school-age children, but teenage parents with younger children could enrol on the scheme to receive help with searching for a job and finding and funding training opportunities and child care.

Being a teenage parent

Many teenage mothers live in poverty; 90% of teenage mothers live on benefit.[1]

Around 75% of 15- to 16-year-old mothers remain in their parental home, whereas around 50% of 17- to 18-year-olds live independently. Teenage parents are likely to be housed by the local authority on large estates distant from their family or other sources of support. Some of them live in supported accommodation such as mother-and-baby hostels, where help with adjusting to parenthood is provided. Young parents who are leaving care to live in their own flat with a young baby are particularly vulnerable to the absence of adult support, and their babies in turn are more likely to be taken into care.[1]

Various studies have reported the likelihood of teenage parents' relationships breaking down.[1] One study found that only about 50% of teenage parents were still together one year after the birth, the rest usually being single and without a regular partner.[4]

Depression is more common in teenage mothers, and occurs in 40% of them within one year of giving birth.[1] Stress arising from conflicts with others, worries about child care and anxiety about making ends meet is common.

The health and development of teenage mothers and their children are improved by promoting access to antenatal care, arranging support by social workers and health visitors, and providing educational opportunities for the mother and pre-school education for the child or children.[5]

Babies of teenage mothers[1]

Teenage mothers have lower birthweight babies and higher infant mortality rates compared to older mothers. These adverse consequences are partly due to the high proportion of pregnant teenage girls who are smokers, and their relatively poor nutrition.

The infant mortality rate for babies of teenage mothers during the first year of life is 60% higher than the rate for babies of older mothers.

Teenage mothers often find parenting far more difficult than they expected. Their children have accidents more often than do children as a whole, and are more likely to be admitted to hospital as a result of an accident (e.g. poisoning or burns) or with gastroenteritis.[1]

Teenage mothers are significantly less likely to breastfeed compared to older mothers, and the children of teenage parents are more likely to live in poverty in poor housing and have poor nutrition.

References

1   Social Exclusion Unit (1999) *Teenage Pregnancy*. The Stationery Office, London.

2   Henderson L (1999) A survey of teenage pregnant women and their male partners in the Grampian region. *Br J Fam Plan.* **25**: 90–92.

3   Chambers R and Milsom G (1995) *Audit of Contraceptive Services in Mid and North Staffordshire in Secondary Care, Primary Care and the Community*. Keele University, Keele.

4   Allen I and Bourke Dowling S (1998) *Teenage Mothers: decisions and outcomes*. Policy Studies Institute, London.

5   NHS Centre for Reviews and Dissemination (1997) Preventing and reducing the adverse effects of unintended teenage pregnancies. *Effect Health Care Bull.* **3**: 1–12.

► CHAPTER 8

Unplanned pregnancy in teenagers

What an unplanned pregnancy means for the woman

An unplanned pregnancy is a disturbing and emotional experience, however much this may be hidden by bravado or blanking it out. Healthcare workers must put aside assumptions that the woman has been foolish, unlucky or careless.

Pregnancy may mean that:

- contraception has failed
- contraception was not used because the woman did not consider herself to be at risk
- the woman did not think that she would be fertile
- she wanted to test out her fertility as 'accidents' previously had not resulted in pregnancy
- she originally wanted to become pregnant, but her circumstances have now changed and she feels it is no longer possible or appropriate
- she is happy to be pregnant but had not planned it
- she does not want to be pregnant but her partner is happy about it
- she is glad to be pregnant but her partner is not happy about it

- she has such a chaotic lifestyle that planning anything is impossible
- it is the result of rape or coercion
- the woman has no other aspirations for the future, so she feels she might as well be pregnant as do anything else
- there are other hidden or open agendas (e.g. the manipulation of circumstances or other people).

The woman needs to be able to discuss what the pregnancy means for her. She will often have mixed feelings and need time to make a decision about what to do. Feeling vulnerable and confused, she may well ask for advice ('What do you think I should do?' or 'What would you do if you were me?'), and it is essential to present the pros and cons of the different options in an unbiased way so that she can reach her *own* decision.

L had just had her fifteenth birthday and had missed two periods. She had only had intercourse a few times with a partner and then the relationship had ended. She was tearful and emotional when she was told that the pregnancy test was positive. She said that she could not have an abortion as she did not 'believe in them'. The GP started arrangements for her antenatal care. Two days later L was back with her mother. L had now decided on a termination. There were more discussions and a referral was made for a termination appointment. L failed to keep that appointment. The midwife visited her at home to arrange antenatal care. Following this, L attended requesting referral for termination. She was calm and determined that this was what she now wanted. She had had a 'chance to think it all through' and could see that a baby at this stage of her life would be a disaster. She had thought that she would like to be a mother herself or that her own mother would look after the baby, but she had

continued

not thought about how she would manage practically in any detail. Talking to the midwife about what was involved had made her realise the full extent of her problems. The pressure from her mother to have a termination had initially made her more determined to do her own thing, but now she had decided for herself.

Pregnancy testing

The first task for the healthcare worker is to establish the facts. The date of the last menstrual period (LMP) is often vague or even completely unknown. If in doubt, *test*. Modern pregnancy tests are highly sensitive to small increases in hormone levels and are usually reliable a few days after the expected but missed period. If the dates are unknown and the test is negative, it may be necessary to re-test one or two weeks later (having advised the woman about contraceptive precautions in the mean time).

Make sure that you know the policy for pregnancy tests in your workplace. If the woman has already done a home test that was positive, she may be offended and think that you disbelieve her if you repeat the test without giving an explanation.

If you are unable to perform a pregnancy test immediately, discuss with the woman how quickly the result is needed. Advise her on alternative ways of obtaining a test result more rapidly (e.g. from a chemist or a clinic), any cost involved, and what she should do when she has the result.

Consider carefully how to give someone their pregnancy test result. Tears of anger (at being stupid, at a partner, about failing others, at health professionals or just at life) may result, and should be allowed to flow with a box of tissues ready to hand. If there is a stunned silence this should be respected, and inappropriate laughter or a light-hearted response recognised for its defensiveness. Only once the immediate emotional response has been expressed can rational thought begin about

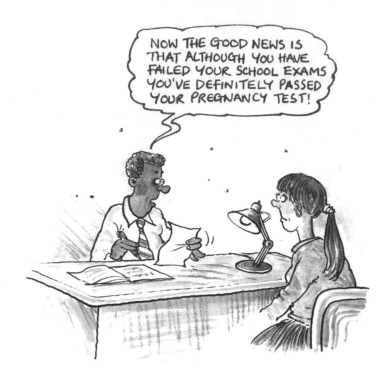

what to do next. This may not occur at the same attendance, and the woman may want time to go away and think about the situation before discussing it any further. Even if she has come prepared with a decision, it is always appropriate to offer another appointment, as factors that were not previously considered may emerge later.

Personal and professional responsibility for health professionals

It is essential to remember that it is not the job of the health professional to tell the woman what she should do, whatever her age. Professional responsibility means that you are entitled to your own views and feelings, but these should not influence or inhibit your treatment of others. There may be circumstances in which you as an individual should opt out of giving information, because your own emotional state is not sufficiently under control to prevent bias. For example, if you have recently had a miscarriage or a bereavement or if you are personally involved in fertility investigations or treatment, it would be expecting too much of yourself to remain detached.

Similarly, if you have strong religious or personal objections to abortion, motherhood outside marriage or young girls having babies, you should arrange for another person to counsel the patient without delay. You may wish to print information about your views, and where else the patient can attend, in the practice leaflet or make this clear to the other members of staff with whom you work.

Decision making about unwanted pregnancy

The degree of distress and confusion experienced by women coping with an unplanned pregnancy varies greatly, but nearly everyone welcomes the chance to talk about their feelings.

Some women will prefer to seek out a healthcare worker previously unknown to them, because they feel that they cannot be advised by or confide in someone they know. They may not want their regular doctor or practice nurse to know that they are pregnant, because they are blaming themselves and fear that others will also blame them. Access to counselling services varies widely in different areas, but if there are charitable agencies or clinics in your area, do not feel rejected if young pregnant women prefer to see a stranger who may be of more help to them at such a critical time.

Some women will opt to continue with the pregnancy and wish to have a baby. They should be made aware of the support services available (*see* Chapter 7 on pregnancy) and have a clear idea of the pros and cons of their decision. A useful self-help book for teenagers working through their decision is available from the National Children's Bureau.[1]

Fostering and adoption are options that have been chosen less often since the Abortion Act became law. Sometimes a woman may decide that she cannot care for a child but that she also cannot have an abortion. She then needs to be put in touch with social workers and child-care and legal advisers, so that she can make an appropriate decision after she knows all the facts. She may also need support from a voluntary organisation, especially if there is opposition to her decision from her family or a partner.

The woman may choose to have an abortion. However much the health professional may hope that she will make a speedy decision about this, it is important that the woman herself takes enough time to make a considered decision. Once the pregnancy has been terminated she cannot change her mind. If she is in any doubt, then she must be offered more time and perhaps more specialised counselling. Not making a decision may be the woman's way of indicating that she does not want to have the pregnancy terminated.

Once her decision has been made, the referral from primary to secondary care should be made quickly.

The legal aspects of abortion

The Abortion Act (1967) made abortion legal under certain specified conditions.

1 The continuance of the pregnancy would involve risk to the life of the pregnant woman greater than if the pregnancy was to be terminated.
2 The continuance of the pregnancy would involve risk of injury to the physical or mental health of the pregnant woman greater than if the pregnancy was to be terminated.
3 The continuance of the pregnancy would involve risk of injury to the physical or mental health of the existing child(ren) of the family of the woman greater than if the pregnancy was to be terminated.

4 There is a substantial risk that if the child was born it would suffer from such physical or mental abnormalities as to be seriously handicapped.

No specific time limits were included in this original Act, and the provisions of the Infant Life Preservation Act of 1929 still applied (that it was illegal to abort a viable pregnancy). Viability was defined in this Act as after week 28 of pregnancy, so abortion had to be carried out before week 28.

The Abortion Act was amended by the Human Fertilisation and Embryology Act (1990), which recognised that advances in medical treatment had enabled viability to be redefined. The amendments changed the Act to include:

1 a new time limit for abortion set at 24 weeks
2 a removal of the time limit of 28 weeks in the Infant Life Preservation Act for specific circumstances where there was considered to be risk:

- to the life of the pregnant woman
- of permanent damage to the mental or physical health of the woman
- that the child would be seriously handicapped.

Two medical practitioners need to agree that the criteria of the Abortion Act have been fulfilled.

Public opinion about abortion

The opponents of legalised abortion believe that it is ethically or morally wrong. However, making abortion illegal does not prevent women from seeking it, and illegal abortion killed or harmed many women before abortion was made legal.[2] Countries where previous legal abortion laws have been removed have shown large increases in morbidity and mortality during the reproductive years. According to the Confidential Enquiries into Maternal Deaths,[3] there were 77 deaths due to illegal abortion in England and Wales in 1961–63, one death in

1979–81 and none since then. Between 1991 and 1993, five deaths due to legal abortion were recorded in the UK.

In a 1997 MORI poll,[4] 64% of those questioned agreed that 'abortion should be made legally available for all those who want it'. Another MORI poll in the previous year revealed that 59% of people questioned did not know that the law required a woman to secure the permission of two doctors before an abortion could be performed, and 53% supported a change to make abortion available on request during the first three months of pregnancy.

Special considerations for teenagers under 16-years-old

The wishes of the young woman must be paramount, but it may take more effort to help her to understand the consequences of the pregnancy and the options open to her. During this time her right to confidentiality must be respected, unless there are overwhelming reasons for a breach (e.g. because of rape or sexual abuse) (*see* Chapter 5 on confidentiality).

A young woman under 16 years of age may consent to abortion without parental knowledge if both of the doctors agree that she has sufficient maturity and understanding to appreciate what is involved. In practice, most doctors would prefer to have the consent or support of a parent or other responsible adult before the procedure is performed.

Young women often present later in pregnancy because of lack of information or because of fear or denial.

The pregnant teenager may wish to try to protect her family from knowing about her sexuality or may even deny to herself that she has been sexually active.

W came with her mother to see her GP. She had been vomiting and feeling sick for over a week. She was 14 years

continued

of age and looked younger. The doctor had some difficulty both in getting her to talk and then in arranging that her mother did not accompany them into the examination room. Enquiries about periods were met with insistence from the girl that she was 'not like that' and that she had not missed a period. A check for diabetes was negative. One week later W was still vomiting and had fainted at school that day. The doctor asked the mother what she thought was wrong. The mother hesitated and then asked if a pregnancy test could be done. W said she didn't need one. The doctor spent some time trying to persuade W to put her mother's and the doctor's minds at rest by having a test. W remained adamant, but later a urine specimen arrived with a note from her mother stating that she had persuaded her. It was positive. Still W denied having been at risk, even after an ultrasound scan confirmed that she was eight weeks pregnant.

The woman may feel isolated from her peer group and unable to use the support network of friends and family. Follow-up appointments in general practice or with a contraceptive service may help her to come to terms with her emotional response.

Many health professionals will have children of a similar age and may find it particularly difficult to deal objectively with a pregnant 14- or 15-year-old. They should recognise their difficulties and refer these young people on to others if they cannot avoid bias or pressure because of their personal feelings.

Abortion procedures

The fact that unprotected intercourse has taken place means that infection may also be present. Screening for infection, especially for the identification of chlamydia, is normally carried out. Contact tracing should be attempted if chlamydia or other infection is found. Treatment should be started before the abortion in order to prevent ascending infection possibly compromising fertility later.

The patient's blood group must be established so that Anti-D can be given to Rhesus-negative women, and general screening for anaemia is normally performed at the same time.

The general health of young women in the UK is usually good, but it is sensible to establish whether any problems exist prior to the procedure, especially if the referral has not come from the woman's general practitioner.

Medical termination of pregnancy (MTOP)

This method is becoming increasingly widely available, especially through the more specialised charitable, private or dedicated NHS clinics. In 1997, 6.6% of abortions were performed by this method.

The woman must be a non-smoker, fit and healthy, and less than 63 days must have elapsed since her last menstrual period. After the initial consultation and screening, the woman takes three tablets of mifepristone, and is then able to go home and resume her normal activities. Two days later she returns to the clinic or hospital and a vaginal pessary of prostaglandin is inserted. This usually results in complete expulsion of the uterine contents within four to six hours. About 5% of women require surgical removal of the remaining contents, and about one-third experience severe cramping after insertion of the prostaglandin pessary. Some women find the procedure distressing, while others prefer to feel in control of the process and are glad to be able to avoid a general anaesthetic.

Suction termination of pregnancy (STOP)

A suction termination of pregnancy is usually offered for a pregnancy that is under 12 weeks gestation. It can be performed under local cervical anaesthesia (up to about 9 weeks gestation) or under a general anaesthetic (this is more usual in the UK). STOP is usually undertaken as a day case. The woman is admitted to hospital having had nothing to eat or drink for at least six hours. After anaesthesia, the cervical canal is dilated and vacuum aspiration is used to remove the uterine contents. This takes about 10 minutes and there should only be mild uterine cramp or discomfort. The bleeding that follows should be like a normal period.

Women should be warned of the possible complications which may occur, as they will normally be discharged from hospital or the clinic after about four hours. Heavy, prolonged or very painful bleeding, especially with a rise in temperature, may indicate infection or incomplete removal of the products of conception. Abdominal pain could suggest a perforation of the uterus (possible although rare). Arrangements for obtaining medical help in such cases should be clear, and preferably backed up with written information, especially if a general anaesthetic has been given.

Most women feel up to carrying out their normal physical activities after 48 hours, but emotional recovery often takes longer.

Mid-trimester and late abortion

Mid-trimester abortions that take place between 13 and 18 weeks gestation are increasingly common the younger the woman. Less than 5% of abortions are performed after 19 weeks, and these are usually carried out because of severe foetal abnormalities.[5] Reasons for terminations being performed after 12 weeks include personal factors such as:

- ignorance about where or how to seek help
- fear or embarrassment about seeking help
- denial of pregnancy
- bleeding in early pregnancy being interpreted as menstrual loss.

Other external factors that may be the reason for termination include:

- lack of access to medical services
- delay in obtaining a pregnancy test result
- delay in obtaining a consultation with a doctor
- unhelpful or biased doctors who delay or refuse referral
- poor or inadequate local provision for terminations causing delay
- antenatal screening detecting abnormalities late in pregnancy
- recent information about health risks to the woman (e.g. a positive HIV test).

Physical complications after abortion increase after 15 weeks gestation, and vacuum extraction is not usually possible by this stage.

Prostaglandin abortion

Vaginal pessaries or an intravenous infusion of prostaglandin are given, which cause evacuation of the uterine contents. Most women complete this process within 12 to 20 hours and require analgesics for the cramp-like contractions. Following this, the woman has a dilatation and curettage under general anaesthesia to ensure that all of the products of conception are removed. A two-day stay in hospital is usual, and this may be difficult to manage in a specialised clinic some distance from home. Patients may encounter a resentful atmosphere in a general gynaecological ward, where other women are being cared for after spontaneous and regretted miscarriages or with infertility or serious gynaecological conditions.

Dilatation and evacuation

This procedure, which is performed under general anaesthesia, is less distressing for the woman, but more difficult both physically and emotionally for the surgeon and his or her assistants. The cervical canal is dilated and the contents of the uterus are removed piecemeal. Complications may include infection, failure to remove all of the products of conception or perforation of the uterus. The stretching of the cervical canal can damage the cervix and lead to cervical incompetence, increasing the risk of miscarriage in subsequent pregnancies.

Contraception

Many young women state that they will never have sex again after discovering that they have an unwanted pregnancy. This is very unlikely! After a decision has been made about the unwanted pregnancy, future plans should always be discussed. After termination during the first 12 weeks contraception can be started *immediately*, whatever the choice of method.

A mid-trimester abortion should be treated in the same way as a delivery, as there is possibly a higher risk of thrombosis. Bleeding problems are also more likely than after a first-trimester termination. Combined oral contraceptives can be started once the patient is fully mobile or at 21 days after a mid-trimester termination. Injectable contraceptives are probably best started or an intrauterine device inserted after 6 weeks, unless the risk of pregnancy before then is high. It is important to help the woman to make a decision based on her own wishes and her risk assessment.

Follow-up after termination

Many women default from follow-up appointments after termination. This is often due to the fact that they wish to forget about the whole business or blank it out and pretend that it did not happen.

Other women are glad of the opportunity to discuss how they now feel about it, and to check that they are physically back to normal. Women who have had a termination often fear that the experience may somehow have damaged their physical body in the same way that they feel their psychological state has been affected.

You should make follow-up arrangements in co-operation with the wishes of the young woman. She will usually find it difficult to return to the place where the termination was performed, and will prefer to return to the clinic or doctor who referred her. People's reactions to the experience vary enormously, from relief that it is over and they can get on with their life to a prolonged period of mourning despite having chosen that course of action. Unresolved feelings sometimes emerge later on (e.g. with another pregnancy, a birth or a subsequent illness).

Contraceptive problems may be an indicator of unresolved feelings. The patient who wants repeated pregnancy tests while experiencing amenorrhoea due to injectable progestogen contraception, or who examines every condom for damage after use, needs help to examine her fears. The woman who frequently forgets her pills, or who has repeated emergency contraception after unprotected intercourse, may unconsciously be testing out her fertility after what she perceives to have been a damaging experience.

Fortunately, most young women recover from the experience of having a termination with the resilience that they show after other adverse events. It is important for the health professional not to ascribe too much significance to an event just because of their own personal feelings.

Charitable abortion resources

British Pregnancy Advisory Services. *Tel*: 01564 793225. Provides details of local branches.

Marie Stopes (London, *Tel*: 020 7388 2585; Leeds, *Tel*: 01132 440685; Manchester, *Tel*: 0161 832 4260).

Counselling and advisory services

Abortion Anonymous. *Tel*: 020 7350 2229. A free telephone counselling service.

Brook Advisory Services. *Tel*: 020 7713 9000. Provides details of local clinics nationwide that provide contraception, pregnancy testing, abortion advice and counselling.

References

1 Mason J and Lewis H (1999) *Time to Decide: a guide for young people in public care when making decisions about pregnancy*. National Children's Bureau, London.

2 Francome C (1977) Estimating the number of illegal abortions. *J Biosoc Sci*. **9**: 467–79.

3 Department of Health (1996) *Report on Confidential Enquiries Into Maternal Deaths in the United Kingdom 1991–93*. HMSO, London.

4 MORI (1997) *Public Attitudes to Abortion*. Birth Control Trust, London.

5 Office for National Statistics (2000) *Population Trends 99*. Government Statistical Service, The Stationery Office, London.

► CHAPTER 9

Misconceptions and myths

Anyone who has incorrect information is at a disadvantage. In the belief that they have the necessary knowledge they do not seek out further information. The knowledge that they do have may lead them to take unnecessary risks or expose them to other harmful effects.

Some of the misunderstandings or misinterpretations that can affect people's sexual lives are discussed below. These include ideas that are prevalent among young people, as well as beliefs that are due to out-of-date medical knowledge or misunderstandings of the way in which fertility or fertility control works.

First, let us dispel the myth that sex education has caused unwanted pregnancies and earlier sexual activity. The World Health Organization examined 19 studies and concluded that sex and HIV/AIDS education does not promote earlier or increased sexual activity in young people. In fact, such education leads to a greater uptake of safer sexual practices.[1] In the UK, school sex education is still treated warily and depends very much on the attitudes of the governors and staff in individual schools. Numerous surveys of young people have concluded that they receive too little information and often too late. Fifteen years ago, pregnancy rates across Europe were very similar, but studies have shown that teenage pregnancy rates have subsequently fallen, particularly in The Netherlands, Sweden and Denmark[2] (*see* Chapter 1). These countries have effective sex education programmes and contraceptive services for young people, and discussion of sexual activity is much more open than in the UK. They have much lower teenage pregnancy rates than does the UK, and their teenagers delay sexual activity to a later age than in the UK.[3]

Common myths about sexual activity in the UK

Many teenagers worry if they are still virgins at 15, 16 or 17 years of age. They tend to believe that everyone is sexually active except them. In the National Survey of Sexual Attitudes and Lifestyles,[4] 19% of female teenagers and 28% of males currently aged 16–19 years reported that they had their first sexual intercourse before the age of 16 years. Thus over 80% of girls and nearly 75% of boys did *not* have sexual intercourse before the age of 16 years. Unfortunately, if adults tell them this, they do not believe it – they tend only to accept such information if it comes from their own peer group. With acute perception they see that adults would prefer them not to be sexually active, and they believe that this information is part of the plot to control their sexuality. To admit to being a virgin, or even to wanting to remain one, appears to be unacceptable and does not conform to the norms of their peer group. Therefore young people pretend they are sexually active and lie about their experiences, even to the point of taking contraceptives which they do not need.

Other beliefs that cause difficulties – and not just in the teenage years – are that all physical contact must lead to sex, that sex must involve penetration, that a man is always ready to have sex, and that a man should not express emotions such as tenderness. These ideas lead to the view that sexual activity is about 'getting notches on your gun' or having sex with as many different partners as possible.

Adolescent teenagers who present at young people's clinics often want to talk about the burden that they feel about beginning relationships.

J attends a clinic in order to obtain some condoms. He is very anxious and asks if the nurse can give him some advice. Should he try for sex on a first date, and if he does not will the girl think he is 'not a man' or even that he is homosexual? If not on the first date, when should he make the move, and how will he know whether the girl wants to have sex? What if he is no good at it and she laughs at him or, worse still, tells all his friends?

There is still pressure on young men to initiate sex, and to believe that it is the performance that counts, not the person or how well you get on together. It is not surprising therefore that so many young teenagers are disappointed by their early sexual encounters, especially when both partners are inexperienced. They are unaware that it takes time and practice to perform well at any skill, including sexual intercourse.

Many of the Victorian ideas about the differences between men and women still exist, and they are often perpetuated in magazines. It is still possible to read articles about 'how to satisfy your man', and others implying that women do not enjoy sex as much as men. It is suggested that men prefer inhibited women or that they feel threatened if the woman takes the lead. Of course, some men do feel threatened in this situation, but others will find it more arousing. Generalisations about people's sexuality are not useful for individual couples. Teenage girls usually worry about what a boy will think of them if they prepare for sexual activity by going on the pill or carrying condoms. Will the boy think they are too forward, not a 'nice' girl or ready to have sex with just anyone? Will they get a reputation for being too 'easy'?

A more dangerous myth, that women say 'No' when they mean 'Yes', is not just believed by ageing judges, but is still held to be true by a (thankfully small) minority of men. These attitudes can lead to date rape or at the very least to coercive sexual intercourse.

The belief that exciting sex involves risk, or that sex should always be natural and spontaneous, often results in lack of use of contraception. If you believe that sexual intercourse should be the sequel to being swept off your feet in a turmoil of passion, you can hardly plan contraception in advance! Disappointment often follows such encounters, and what many teenagers who attend for emergency contraception say about their sexual experiences is that they felt let down or cheated by the lack of feeling.

Two girls attended the young people's clinic for emergency contraception. They do everything together and therefore wanted to see the doctor together. It was the first time for them both. They were at a party with some boys whom they knew. They chorused that it had not been a big deal – they couldn't see what all the fuss was about and did not want to do 'it' again. Now they wished that they had gone home earlier and avoided the situation altogether. Then one of them said 'Well, at least I'm not a virgin any more, so I don't have to worry about that'.

The attitude that sex is a subject that is not talked about (or if it is, only referred to by innuendo and embarrassed laughter) is taking a long time to disappear from the UK. The view that 'if you don't mention sex, teenagers will not be interested in it' has been disproved over and over again. If you have no experience of talking about sexual activity at home in an open and matter-of-fact way, you are more likely to find it difficult to negotiate the use of a condom when starting sexual intercourse with a new partner. If you cannot talk about sex, how will you know when to start on contraception or where to obtain it? Of course, prurient interest in the details of young people's sexual activity is almost as offputting – sexual activity is private and the relationship something to be valued and respected. However, if a parent or guardian does not ask if contraception is needed or whether it has been considered, this is likely to lead to the absence of contraception and the presence of an unwanted pregnancy instead.

False beliefs are common. Steph Chambers has collected some of the most common ones (*see* final section of this chapter) and others are described below.

False beliefs about getting pregnant

Unfortunately, obtaining information from your friends, rather than from trained professionals or from accurate books,

Table 9.1: Some commonly held false beliefs about getting pregnant

False idea	Reality
You can't get pregnant:	
If you do it twice in a row or one day after another; the second time you don't need a condom because there are no sperm left	*Each* ejaculate contains over 300 million sperm
If you are not doing it often	You are *less* likely to become pregnant, but still running a risk
If you don't have an orgasm	Orgasm is not necessary to draw the sperm into the uterus – they swim quite well without!
If he's been doing it for ages and not got anyone pregnant yet	Intercourse with someone else is no guarantee for this relationship
If he presses in the groin before ejaculating; this prevents the sperm from getting out	The sperm are already in the seminal vesicles in the prostate gland long before orgasm is imminent

can result in an unwanted pregnancy. The stories that are bandied about (*see* Table 9.1) are often the result of wishful thinking or sometimes plain falsehood for sexual gain.

False ideas about contraception

Again misinformation obtained from friends or from confused or biased newspaper reports can lead to pregnancy (*see* Table 9.2). Sometimes false information is given by people who think that they know about the subject, but their knowledge is inaccurate or out of date.

Table 9.2: Some commonly held false beliefs about contraception

False idea	Reality
Withdrawal is useless	It is better than nothing, but must be backed up with emergency contraception
It is easy to work out when you will be fertile by counting 14 days from the first day of your last period	Ovulation occurs about 14 days before the *next* period. Few women have absolutely regular 28-day cycles, and illness or other events, including the use of emergency contraception, may delay the next period. Sperm live for up to 7 days in the genital tract, but the egg can only be fertilised up to about 12 hours after release
You cannot be given contraception until you are 16-years-old	Being under 16-years-old is no protection against becoming pregnant, and teenagers below this age can be given contraception (*see* Chapter 6 on contraception and Chapter 5 on confidentiality)
Every tenth condom has a hole in it	Condoms with a kite mark (BSI-tested) are safe
Condoms burst easily	Have you ever tried blowing one up? However, they do tear, on fingernails, rings or because of friction

Fears and misunderstandings about the pill and injections

Aren't oral contraceptives risky?

The simple answer to this question is that the pill is less risky than a pregnancy in any healthy young woman. The reason for taking a history is to establish the few contra-indications to using oestrogen-containing pills. Even in these women (e.g. those with severe migraine) progestogen-only methods can often be considered.

The risks associated with smoking (a common practice among many adolescents) are much higher than the risks linked with either being pregnant or taking oral contraceptives.

Heart attacks

Women who do not smoke and do not have any other risk factors for cardiac disease are at little if any extra risk of myocardial infarction if they take the pill. The relative risk of a myocardial infarction is 20 times higher in women who smoke more than 15 cigarettes daily and use the combined oral contraceptive pill, compared to non-pill users who do not smoke. However, the risk of heart attacks in young women is very low.

Venous thrombosis

Venous thrombosis associated with oestrogen use may occur in higher-risk women. It must be explained that this is not a risk to life in itself, but only if it causes part of a clot to break off and travel to another part of the body (thromboembolism).

The family history, if known, may be useful for predicting the likelihood of thromboembolism, but more than 50% of individuals who develop venous thromboembolism (VTE) have no detectable hereditary defects of coagulation.

Figures from the World Health Organization Scientific Group[5] give a background risk for VTE of 5 per 100 000 women per year, 60 per 100 000 pregnancies and 15 per 100 000 women per year for second-generation combined oral contraceptives (COCs). The media attention surrounding the publication of evidence in 1995 which showed an increased risk of VTE of 25–30 per 100 000 women per year using third-generation COCs caused many women to stop taking the pill and thus be exposed to a greater risk of VTE due to pregnancy.

Clots that occur in the menstrual loss are *not* associated with any increased risk, nor are they associated with thrombosis in any way.

No-one should be diagnosed as having a deep venous thrombosis in the leg on the basis of leg pain or cramp alone. If there is pain in only one leg, then COCs should be stopped (and another method of contraception used) while investigations are carried out. A woman's future healthcare and contraceptive method both depend on an accurate diagnosis.

Stroke

Research published by the World Health Organization[6] emphasises the importance of a raised blood pressure and smoking in the aetiology of stroke. Haemorrhagic stroke is increased by both of these factors but not by the use of COCs. Ischaemic stroke is related to thrombosis and is increased in COC users, but the risk increases markedly in smokers. Although haemorrhagic stroke can occur at any age (though the incidence increases with age), ischaemic stroke is extremely rare in young people, and the increased risk was reported for individuals over 35 years of age.

Fears about weight gain

One of the major concerns of young women is about weight gain. Most teenagers compare themselves with the models they see illustrated in magazines or on television. The normal change in body shape (especially the development of hips and fatter thighs) that occurs in adolescence is often misinterpreted as being 'gross' and 'fat'.

Weight gain is often blamed on the pill, and even when it can be demonstrated that no change in weight has occurred, the change in shape is too much to bear. Most studies of COCs show that 60% of women who are on the pill do not show any significant change in weight, which varies between ± 2 kilograms. About 20–25% of women on the pill will gain more than that, and 15–20% will lose more than that. Of course, the steady increase in weight that occurs during adolescence also has to be taken into account.

Counselling before starting injectable progestogens is important, as most women gain some weight, usually about 2 kilograms in the first year. A few women seem to put on weight very rapidly. However, increased appetite appears to be the main cause, rather than fluid retention.

Fears about fertility

It used to be common practice to have regular breaks off the COC every few years. In fact, all that happened was that women were at higher risk of pregnancy while using a less efficient method, and often manifested this with an unplanned pregnancy.

Indeed, the COC does much to *reduce* the risks of infertility. There is a lower risk of pelvic infection, fewer ectopic pregnancies, less endometriosis, and less risk of functional ovarian cysts, all of which may impair future fertility due to the presence of pelvic adhesions, scarring or surgical interference. Thus there is no rational reason for having breaks from the COC or worrying about fertility – at least not until well past the teenage years, when age alone may impair fertility.

Many teenagers express fears that having the progestogen injection will make them 'sterile'. This is partly due to muddled thinking about the purpose of regular menstruation, and partly due to fears about stories they have heard of women taking a long time to become pregnant after stopping the injection. The absence of the menstrual cycle does usually imply inability to become pregnant – but not permanently, only until ovulation is re-established, which is usually about 14 days before the next menses occurs. After use of progestogen injections there may be a delay before full fertility is restored. In a large study of women in Thailand[7] who discontinued progestogen injections, the mean time to conception was nine months, and by two years fertility rates were normal compared to users of other methods of contraception. The restoration of fertility is often quicker than this, particularly in underweight women, so the delay in restoration of fertility should not be relied upon if pregnancy is undesirable!

Fears about cancer

Breast cancer seems to be a particular cause for concern, which is often out of proportion to the actual risk. A recognised risk factor for breast cancer is late age at the time of the first full-term pregnancy – and the pill or injection delays pregnancy very effectively. The risk of breast cancer in young women is very small (1 in 500 up to the age of 35 years), so an increase in the risk will result in very small numbers of sufferers. Current pill-users experience an increase of about 25% in this very small risk, but this wanes in ex-users and is not detectable 10 years after use.[8]

Tenderness of the breast after starting hormonal contraception is *not* a sign that the woman will develop cancer later. Increases in the incidence of breast cancer, cervical cancer and the very rare liver tumours need to be balanced against the reduction in rates of uterine and ovarian cancer that occur in women using hormonal contraception. Overall, the balance is probably about equal. Currently available hormonal contraceptives do not appear to be associated with a net excess risk.[9] The facts about the beneficial effects of COCs (*see* Table 9.3) are often lost amidst the media-induced hysteria. The COC provides excellent contraception as well, so preventing the complications of childbirth.

Table 9.3: Potential health benefits of combined oral contraceptive pills

Medical condition	Reduction in risk of medical condition
Iron-deficiency anaemia	Reduced amount of loss during menses
Pelvic inflammatory disease	50%
Ectopic pregnancy	90%
Benign breast disease	50–70%
Retention cysts of the ovary	From 38 per million women to 3 per million
Endometrial cancer	50%
Ovarian cancer	40%
Dysmenorrhoea	Especially if associated with heavy menses
Premenstrual syndrome	Can reduce the hormonal fluctuations
Fibroids	30%
Peptic ulcer	Only slight evidence
Rheumatoid arthritis	Some studies have shown a reduction in incidence or slowing of disease progression; other studies have not
Thyroid disease	Less common according to a large Royal College of General Practitioners study[9]

Miscellaneous myths

'*Women get more drunk if they are on the pill.*' There are conflicting views about this. One report suggests that alcohol is cleared more slowly in COC users, and another suggests that women recover more quickly! It is wise advice to women on the pill not to drink too much – they may have sex unwisely or vomit after taking their pill, both of which put them at risk.

'*Women should not take the pill if they are flying.*' Flying, especially if combined with sitting in a confined space (such as an airline seat), dehydration and the lower oxygen concentration in an aircraft, increases the risk of thrombosis. This risk can be reduced by frequent activity, and consuming adequate amounts of non-alcoholic fluids. Pregnancy (which has a higher risk of thrombosis) should not be risked by stopping the pill.

'*The worst pill to miss is in the middle of the packet.*' This belief has arisen from confusion about the normal menstrual cycle, in which ovulation occurs about mid-cycle, and ovulation is absent if the woman is taking COCs. The worst pill to forget is the first one in the pack, when a break of seven days may have already allowed the ovary to produce a ripening follicle (*see* Chapter 6 on contraception).

'*If you miss a pill or take antibiotics, don't bother to carry on with the pill because it isn't going to work.*' Missing *more* pills makes it *more* likely for ovulation to occur, so the pill should be continued in order to send the ovaries back to sleep!

'*The pill gives you spots.*' If acne becomes worse or appears for the first time while taking the pill, then a change of type of COC is needed, as some women are more sensitive to the effects of progestogens than others.

'*My doctor doesn't believe in the injection.*' It is more likely that doctors who do not use the full range of contraceptive methods have less interest in the subject and are less well informed.

'*I couldn't get emergency pills because of the Bank Holiday, so it's too late to do anything. I can't have a coil because I haven't had a baby.*' The woman could still be fitted with an intra-uterine device. These devices *can* be fitted in women who have not had children (*see* Chapter 6 on contraception).

'*I don't want a coil; it will set off the metal detector in airports.*' Fortunately this does not happen.

'*My friend said her coil came out when she and her boyfriend were trying out some new positions.*' There is no evidence that an IUD which is correctly positioned will be expelled during sexual athletics. This will only happen if it is already on its way out.

'*I had the morning-after pill just after my period this month; now we've had another accident, so I won't be able to have it again.*' It can be given again, but the woman should find a more reliable method in the future.

Misconceptions about oral contraceptives are summarised in Table 9.4.

Table 9.4: Misconceptions about oral contraceptives

Don't use the pill if you have:	Reality – are there additional risks?
Worries about future fertility	Fertility is protected by reduced risk of pelvic inflammatory disease, polycystic ovarian syndrome, fibroids, etc.
Worries about birth defects	No excess risk
Breast lumps or fibroids	Reduced risk of benign breast lumps, reduced risk of fibroids
Past amenorrhoea	Neutral, may be beneficial
Recent menarche	Neutral
Varicose veins	Neutral, unless there is a history of thrombophlebitis
Thrush	Neutral
Sickle-cell trait	Neutral
Sickle-cell disease	Use a progestogen injection, as it is protective
Abnormal cervical smear	Use a barrier method as well; have regular screening
Epilepsy	Higher dose necessary
Migraine	Only avoid if it is focal or if it worsens
Pre-eclamptic toxaemia (PET) in pregnancy	Monitor blood pressure in case it was essential hypertension

Myths about infection

You cannot tell whether someone is likely to have an infection simply by looking at them. Anyone who has a sexual relationship can acquire a sexually transmitted disease (STD).

> Dr L was doing his family planning training in a clinic, supervised by an experienced doctor. He saw one 16-year-old who gave a history of having started bleeding while
>
> *continued*

taking her oral contraceptive pill. He discovered that she had been taking it for 18 months without previous problems. She was wearing a very short skirt, long boots and a large amount of eye make-up, and she giggled a great deal in a rather provocative way. He asked about her partners, and she told him that she had just changed partners after being with the previous one 'for ages – about six months'. He talked to her about chlamydia and she gave her consent to vaginal swabs being taken.

Two patients later, an 18-year-old woman came in. She was dressed in a rather smart trouser suit with a name badge on her lapel which said that she was a trainee manager for a large store. She looked professional and wore discreet make-up. She gave a history of bleeding while taking her oral contraceptive. She had been on the same type for 18 months and had not had any problems previously. Dr L had started to talk to her about changing the pill when the supervising doctor coughed and interrupted him to suggest that he recalled how he had talked about chlamydia previously. This patient gave a history of having had three partners in the last 12 months, and she had split up with one of them after discovering he was two-timing her. Dr L obtained consent for vaginal swabs to be taken from this patient as well. After the patient had left, the two doctors discussed how easy it is to make assumptions about a person's lifestyle from their appearance.

Tackling misinformation

If you do not know what people believe, you cannot put those beliefs right when they are wrong. Using open-ended questions such as 'What do you think?' and 'Tell me what you know already' often helps to identify where the problems lie.

Checking that a woman knows how to take the oral contraceptive pill is not just a matter of saying 'do you understand what to do?' but of asking her to run through what she is going to do. If she can tell you this correctly, it is likely that she has understood. Always give plenty of opportunity for answers to the question 'Is there anything else you wanted to ask about?'. 'Not really' may mean that the patient is not sure whether or not to ask, rather than that there is nothing they want to know.

Always be tactful. Your patient will never tell you anything again if you almost fall off your chair laughing at their faulty information or strange ideas. The way in which other people think and reason from the facts that they have available is fascinating. If you think about how the misconception has arisen, it (usually) becomes more understandable. Explain in simple terms how the misunderstanding came about and correct it. Then check that the new reasoning is understood! Be open to other ideas, and do not forget that it might be *your* ideas, beliefs or information that are incorrect. Be prepared to look things up to check that what you think is right is backed up by evidence or at least by authoritative sources.

The patient told the doctor that she only wanted a month's supply of the pill, as she was coming off it to have a baby. The doctor asked why she wanted another month's supply. The patient had just had a rubella injection at work as she had been found on screening not to be immune. 'You have to avoid pregnancy for three months', objected the doctor. The patient was sure that she had been told one month. The doctor looked it up and agreed that the patient was correct.

Keep an open mind and check your information before correcting someone else. We are all fallible.

Myths involving sex – the teenager's perspective

The following contribution from Steph describes the views of her contemporaries

Many teenagers are told myths about sex and getting pregnant. Some of the most common myths are listed below.

'*You can't get pregnant if it's your first time.*'
This myth is one of the most common ones that young people I know do not believe. Nearly all teenagers have heard of this one. Unfortunately, you can get pregnant on your first time just like any other.

'*You can't get pregnant if you have sex standing up.*'
Maybe if magazines and other sources had not educated me otherwise, I might have been susceptible to believing this myth. It seems plausible because you might expect that the sperm could not travel into the uterus because you are standing vertically, but they certainly can.

'*If you have a bath after sex then you can't get pregnant.*'
This is another common myth, and many young people still do believe this because it sounds plausible. They think that bathing will wash all the sperm out of the uterus before they reach the egg. However, it only takes a few seconds for the sperm to reach the egg.

'*You can only take the emergency pill the morning after sex.*'
You can take it 72 hours later but because the hormonal pill has been renamed by most teenagers and many adults, teenagers are led to believe that you can only take this pill *the morning after* having had unprotected sex or, equally, failure of contraception. A high percentage of teenagers do not know that the IUD (intrauterine device) can be fitted as emergency contraception, and they do not know the terms that apply to this use of contraceptives. Not

continued

many of them would know that you can have an IUD fitted up to five days later (or more depending on the stage of the cycle).

'If you use two condoms it will be safer than one.'
To be extra safe many teenagers try wearing two condoms. In theory, this seems to be plausible, but many teenage girls do not know that this may cause friction, and I admit that I too did not realise this fact until I researched this topic.

'I can't fit into a condom.'
This is a common excuse for boys who do not like wearing protection. I am informed by a teenage magazine that condoms are designed to stretch 5 feet and fit all shapes and sizes. Girls believe this myth because they have no way of knowing this fact, unless they have read this particular magazine, and it therefore results in the couple having unprotected sex with the reassuring words 'I'll be careful'. Boys may not know how to put on a condom properly. They may not be applying it properly or leaving a space at the end.

'It's better if you use Vaseline as a lubricant.'
A recent magazine article stated that Vaseline actually dissolves condoms, making them weak in places and more likely to break or become ineffective. Boys do use Vaseline because it is thought to be a good lubricant.

'I'm too young to get you pregnant.'
As soon as boys become sexually active they may be capable of getting someone pregnant. There is not a fixed age, so that any lad aged, say, 15 years or below can't get someone pregnant, yet girls still think that if a boy is young then that means they will not be able to become pregnant.

'I can't get pregnant when I'm just off my period.'
Oh yes she can. It may be slightly less likely, but it is still possible whatever time of the month, but some girls think

continued

that if they are just off their period then they won't have to worry about becoming pregnant. Advice from a site on the Internet reported that 'with a girl's cycle it is practically impossible to say whether she is fertile at that particular moment, or will become fertile within the three days that sperm may stay inside her. The risk of pregnancy from a single act of unprotected mid-cycle intercourse has been estimated at 20–30%.'

Although as a teenager myself I would take everything I find on the Internet with a pinch of salt, I don't know whether what I have read on it to research this topic is true or not, and therefore fall into the trap of believing myths that I'd try to tell young people to ignore. You cannot use the Internet as a reliable source of information, as you cannot see what type of person has set up the site. I am sure it would not be too difficult for someone like myself (an ordinary teenager without any special expert knowledge) to set one up.

'I'll withdraw before I have a chance to let any sperm out.'
This is thought to be an adequate form of contraception among teenagers today. They may try to do this, but it probably won't work completely, and afterwards they may re-enter. Also, as soon as they have an erection they will form a small amount of fluid called pre-ejaculation or pre-cum (also known as 'love drops') which contains sperm. Withdrawal definitely does not work, because no matter how careful you are there are still traces of sperm on the penis.

'It's safe as long as I urinate before and after sex.'
Some males seem to think that urine is a good form of contraception because it leaves an acid lining on the urethra of the penis and this does not let the sperm out. In fact, urine is not a spermicide and this method definitely will not work.

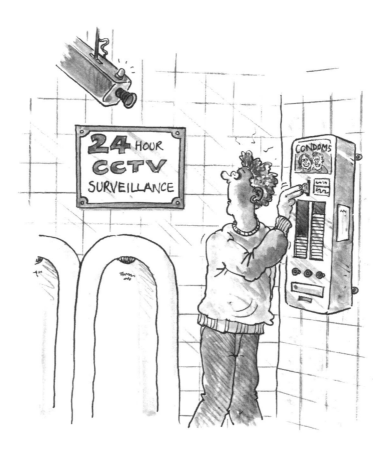

References

1   Baldo M, Aggleton P and Slutkin G (1993) *Does Sex Education Lead to Earlier or Increased Sexual Activity in Youth?* WHO Global Programme on AIDS. World Health Organization, Geneva.

2   Singh S and Darroch JE (2000) Adolescent pregnancy and child-bearing: levels and trends in developed countries. *Fam Plan Perspect.* **32:** 14–23.

3   European Commission (2000) *Report on the State of Young People's Health in the European Union: a Commission Services Working Paper.* European Commission, Brussels.

4   Wellings K, Field J, Johnson AM and Wadsworth J (1994) *Sexual Behaviour in Britain*. Penguin Books, Harmondsworth.

5   World Health Organisation (1988) *Cardiovascular Disease and Steroid Hormone Contraception*. Report of a WHO Scientific Group. World Health Organization, Geneva.

6   World Health Organization Collaborative Group (1996) Ischaemic stroke and combined oral contraceptives: results of an international, multicentre, case-control study. *Lancet*. **348:** 498–505.

7   Pardthaisong T (1984) Return of fertility after use of the injectable contraceptive Depo-Provera: an updated data analysis. *J Biosoc Sci*. **16:** 23–34.

8   Collaborative Group on Hormonal Factors (1996) Breast cancer and hormonal contraceptives: collaborative re-analysis of individual data on 53 297 women with breast cancer and 100 239 women without breast cancer from 54 epidemiological studies. *Lancet*. **347:** 1713–27.

9   Hannaford PC and Kay CR (1998) The risk of serious illness among oral contraceptive users: evidence from the RCGP's oral contraceptive study. *Br J Gen Pract*. **48:** 1657–62.

CHAPTER 10

Sexual diseases and allied problems

What is the problem?

Genito-urinary medicine (GUM) clinics are responsible for making statistical returns to the Department of Health each year of the number of cases of sexually transmitted infections (STIs) seen, categorised by diagnosis and gender. The latest statistics from the Public Health Laboratory Service always lag behind what is currently being seen, and the most recent figures are from 1998.[1] These STI rates from GUM clinics will always be an underestimate, as some cases will be treated in general practice or by other hospital departments (e.g. gynaecology departments) but they are the nearest we can get to assessing what is happening in sexual health. The number of new diagnoses and uptake of services in GUM clinics in 1998 exceeded one million for the first time – 6% higher than in 1997. The Department of Health chose gonorrhoea as a marker of sexual practices in the *Health of the Nation*[2] targets (the target being to reduce the incidence by 20%).

Gonorrhoea cases increased between 1997 and 1998, with the largest rises being reported in London and preliminary data give larger rises still between 1998 and 1999. Those aged between 16 and 19 years were particularly affected, with increases of up to 52% in males and 39% in females.

The rate of identification of chlamydia infections is increasing everywhere. This may be partly due to greater awareness of the significance of chlamydial infection. The number of chlamydia infections in men rose by 17% and in women it increased by 11%. Chlamydial infections are particularly likely to occur in young people under the age of 20 years.

The steepest rise in the first attack of genital warts was found in young men and women aged 16–19 years, and overall the rate increased by 2% from 1997. Infections with herpes simplex virus also increased, but mainly in those over 45 years of age. It is difficult to determine whether STI rates are continuing to rise or whether people are becoming more willing to attend GUM clinics.

What to tell patients about genito-urinary medicine (GUM) clinics

The new name for these clinics causes some confusion. They were previously known as 'special' or 'VD' (venereal disease) clinics or sometimes 'STD' (sexually transmitted disease) clinics – and they have many nicknames, such as the 'clap clinic', 'back-lane' clinic, etc. Access to these clinics varies across the country, and new users often find it difficult to discover what is available. Healthcare workers should know where the GUM clinics are located and how people can be seen. Some clinics have open access, while others require appointments to be made by telephone. Some of them are open in the evening, while others are open from 10 a.m. until 5 p.m. (not very convenient!). Some of the clinics now provide a seamless one-stop service together with contraceptive clinics or are on the same premises to enable easy transfers between the services. Other clinics only provide emergency contraception.

It must be emphasised that the GUM service is confidential. By law the staff cannot tell a patient what infection their partner has or tell their doctor that they have attended, unless the patient requests this. They will record a name and date of birth, and will ask for a contact address, but the patient does not need to give this information if they prefer not to.

At a GUM clinic, tests can be performed immediately to diagnose some infections, while for other tests it will be some time before the results are known. These clinics do need some identifying information so that they can access patients' records when they reattend.

Cervical smears can also be performed, and some clinics can examine the cervix for abnormalities with a colposcope. Some clinics will have sexual problem counsellors or impotence clinics attached to them. All of them have health advisers who can discuss sexual health with clients openly and honestly.

GUM clinics endeavour to be effective in tracing sexual contacts if an infection is present. They may give clients a slip of paper with a coded diagnosis to give to partners or ex-partners, who can then take the slip to *any* GUM clinic and be tested and treated. If clients prefer, the health adviser can contact partners or ex-partners to tell them that they may have been exposed to infection.

How sexually transmitted infections (STIs) present

Patients may present at their general practice or at a clinic with:

- irritation
- painful urination
- discharge from the urethra or vagina
- lumps on the genital area or elsewhere
- ulcers
- pain in the genital area.

Suspicion about the presence of STIs may be raised by finding:

- a raised number of white blood cells (WBCs) with no organisms cultured from the urine
- pelvic pain or dyspareunia

- peri-hepatitis or peri-appendicitis
- menstrual irregularities or intermenstrual bleeding
- cervical smear abnormalities
- miscarriage
- ectopic pregnancy
- premature labour
- conjunctivitis
- reactive arthritis.

The main point is to remember to consider STIs! Everyone who has had sexual contact with a partner is at risk, unless both partners have only ever had contact with each other. Complete monogamy or chastity provides the only (almost) complete protection. The other risks are from non-sexual exchange of body fluids (e.g. needlestick injuries, sharing needles or transmission from mother to infant).

Chlamydia

Chlamydia trachomatis is the most common bacterial STI in the UK. It is frequently without symptoms, and up to 70% of women and 50% of men have the infection unknowingly. Prevalence rates differ widely in various populations – from 1% to 10%[3] – and pilot studies currently being conducted in general practices should help to determine the feasibility of screening. It is an important infection because of its causative role in pelvic inflammatory disease and infertility, ectopic pregnancy and morbidity from chronic pelvic pain. The incidence is increasing, especially in the 16–19 years age group.[1]

Suspicion should be raised in this age group, especially if other risk factors are present such as:

- a recent change of partner
- two or more partners in the last 12 months
- unplanned pregnancy
- bleeding after intercourse or new breakthrough bleeding on oral contraceptives
- dysuria in either sex

- other STI symptoms (e.g. discharge)
- pelvic or abdominal pain
- testicular or epididymal pain.

A cervical (not high vaginal) or urethral swab is needed to obtain cellular material for immunofluorescent testing or else a first-passed specimen of urine if the more expensive but less invasive urine test is available at the laboratory. Treatment is with tetracycline (e.g. doxycycline, 100 mg, twice a day for 7–14 days), erythromycin (500 mg twice a day for 14 days) or a single dose of azithromycin (1 g). Contact tracing should always be attempted, preferably by the GUM clinic.

Gonorrhoea

The incidence of *Neisseria gonorrhoeae* infections is still increasing in the UK. The infection seems to be producing less florid symptoms than in the past, so that many infections are picked up opportunistically. Male symptoms of dysuria, discharge or epididymitis or female symptoms of dysuria, discharge or abdominal pain should raise suspicions. Referral for contact tracing is recommended, and advice on current sensitivities to antibiotics should be obtained from the GUM clinic. It is essential that female contacts, who are often without symptoms, should be treated, particularly as they may suffer long-term adverse effects such as infertility or pelvic infection. Antibiotic resistance is increasing, and high-risk sexual behaviour is also increasing again[4] as the effects of the AIDS/HIV 'safe sex' campaigns are wearing off.

Non-specific urethritis or non-specific genital infection

This is defined as an infection, usually urethritis, that is not caused by gonorrhoea. It is common in young men. Up to 40%

of episodes of urethritis are in fact caused by chlamydia. *Mycoplasma genitalium* and *Ureaplasma urealyticum* are among the other causative organisms. The diagnosis is mainly made on the basis of a combination of symptoms of urethritis and the presence of pus cells (more than 5 pus cells per high-power field at magnification ×400) from an intraurethral swab. The partner(s) should be treated to prevent recurrence. Treatment is as described above for chlamydia.

Trichomonas vaginalis (TV)

Women usually present with an increased vaginal discharge, which may be smelly, frothy and yellowish-green. They may also complain of a sore vagina, painful intercourse and dysuria. A cervical or high vaginal swab usually identifies the organism on microscopy or culture. Men often show no symptoms, but may have dysuria or a penile discharge. It is often difficult to identify the infection from a urethral swab in men. Partners should always be traced to prevent recurrence, and full STI screening is advisable to identify other infections. Treatment is with metronidazole, either as a single dose of 2 g or as a five-day course of 400 mg twice daily.

Two 15-year-old girls from the local Social Services care home arrived giggling at the surgery. They told the practice nurse that they both had a discharge. She tried without success to persuade them to go to the GUM clinic, and referred them to the doctor. After talking it through, they agreed to have swabs taken and to return for the results. They were both worldly wise and fully aware of the consequences of their actions, although they seemed to

continued

care little about the outcome. They both decided to start on the contraceptive pill and take some condoms, as they were at risk, but they refused to give consent for anyone else to be involved. They both had TV infection. Again they refused to attend a GUM clinic or to involve anyone else, but took a number of contact slips to give to their contacts. Over the next few weeks several boys and a few young men turned up at the GUM clinic and the practice with their contact slips. The doctor continued to see both girls frequently to try to give them some support while they sorted out their lifestyle, and to encourage them to be more assertive in their relationships. Unfortunately, both girls left the care home and the area once they were 16-years-old, before much progress had been made.

Genital warts – human papilloma virus (HPV)

The incidence of first-ever presentation of genital warts is increasing, again significantly in the 16–19 years age group.[3]

HPV is common among sexually active young people, whether or not visible warts are present. Genital warts are usually spread sexually, so their presence should prompt a search for other STIs. Some HPVs (types 16, 18, 31 and 34) – not the ones that present as visible warts – are associated with the development of cervical cancer, and more frequent cervical screening is normally suggested if STIs are found. Determining the type of HPV present is still only a research technique at the time of writing. Investigations are in progress to determine the feasibility of using the technique to distinguish between those individuals who require more frequent follow-up and those whose infection is likely to be transient and not associated with a higher risk of cervical cancer. Cervical screening is not usually recommended for women under the age of 20 years, as the cells from an immature cervix may be easily confused with abnormalities, resulting in unnecessary anxiety and extra follow-up.

Herpes simplex (cold sores)

Although it is a less significant infection than other STIs in terms of absolute numbers, herpes causes severe morbidity. The first attack is often extremely painful, sometimes causing retention of urine because of the severe pain as urine passes over the lesions. Recurrent attacks prevent sexual enjoyment and may permanently adversely affect the quality of life, especially if recurrences are frequent. In 1997,[1] 1751 females and 255 males between 16 and 19 years of age were seen in GUM clinics with herpes simplex, and 71 females and three males aged 15 years and 34 females and seven males under 15 years of age had herpes simplex.

Syphilis

New cases of syphilis in the UK are rare, and are mostly found during screening in pregnancy or for blood donation. Referral to a GUM clinic is essential.

Viral hepatitis

Hepatitis B is more infectious than HIV, and can be spread by sexual intercourse as well as from contaminated blood. Immunisation is available to at-risk groups.

Hepatitis A can be transmitted sexually by a partner with an active infection. Immunisation against hepatitis A is now available, either separately or together with hepatitis B.

Human immunodeficiency virus (HIV and AIDS)

New presentations of asymptomatic HIV infection have shown little overall change in the last few years. New presentations of symptomatic HIV and AIDS diagnoses in homosexual men actually decreased by 45% between 1997 and 1998.[1] However, the increase in other STIs suggests that the 'safe sex' message is being forgotten in both homosexual and heterosexual intercourse. The long-term implications of a diagnosis if no symptoms are present have to be considered carefully before a test is performed. The health advisers at GUM clinics are experienced in presenting the risk–benefit ratio to individuals who believe that they may have exposed themselves to risk.

Pubic lice

This infestation commonly coexists with STIs, so screening should be considered.

A 16-year-old student had just arrived back from her exchange with her French penfriend. She asked for assurances that the consultation would not be mentioned to her parents, who did not know she was attending the surgery. She told the doctor that she was very itchy down below and had found some spots of blood on her panties. The doctor asked to examine her and found live lice in the pubic hair. The girl told the doctor that her penfriend was very shocked at some of the places they had ended up exploring together in the town where she lived – she had never dared to go to such places. The doctor was relieved to find that the patient had 'gone on the pill to reduce her heavy periods' before she went to France, but needed to make her an appointment for STI screening before she left the surgery.

Genital infections that are not usually sexually transmitted but easily confused with STIs

Bacterial vaginosis (BV)

This is a common cause of vaginal discharge in primary care. It can create a greyish watery discharge with an offensive fishy smell that develops after intercourse due to the alkaline nature of the ejaculate. It is often found coincidentally. A high vaginal or cervical swab will show the presence of unusual bacteria, often with *Gardnerella vaginalis* and other anaerobic bacteria. Bacterial vaginosis often seems to appear after treatment for other infections. Some authorities have suggested that it is due to replacement of the normal bacterial flora of the vagina following antibiotic treatment or frequent washing. Apart from the aesthetic considerations, there is increasing evidence that preterm deliveries and early pregnancy loss may be associated with BV. Treatment in symptomatic patients or in pregnancy is with metronidazole or clindamycin cream applied locally. The best regime in pregnancy is still under review, and specialist advice should be sought for the current best treatment.

Candida (thrush)

Although this is rarely sexually transmitted, it can be the source of sexual problems. The classic symptoms of a thick creamy discharge and itching with patches of white over red sore vaginal or penile skin are not always seen. *Candida albicans* is an opportunistic infection that exploits lowered immunity, including diabetes, pregnancy, malignancy or HIV infection. The association with antibiotic use for other infections or for acne is more common in teenagers. It can be more frequent in those who carry candida in the gut, and the condition can be helped by giving advice on washing from front to back of the perineum, and avoiding the use of detergents and soap, and local skin damage.

Thrush has not been shown to be associated with the use of low-dose oral contraceptives, and treating the sexual partner rarely reduces the risk of recurrence. Treatment is with local or oral antifungals and prevention or avoidance of precipitating factors.

What is 'safer sex'?

Many people have infections without realising it, and they cannot be identified in advance. The most widely publicised advice has been about avoiding HIV infections, and many young people do not know about the other STIs which they are more likely to catch. A needlestick injury is associated with a 0.3% risk of contracting HIV if it is present, compared to a 30% risk of catching hepatitis B if that infection is present.

The box below summarises the risks of various activities.

The safest sex is no sex – but this may be unrealistic

High risk
- Vaginal or anal intercourse without a condom, including withdrawal (coitus interruptus)
- Giving oral sex to a man and taking the ejaculate into the mouth
- Giving oral sex to a woman during her period (menstruation)
- Unprotected 'rimming' (licking your partner's anal area)
- Finger insertion with cuts or grazes or during menstruation
- Getting human faeces or urine in your mouth
- Sharing sex toys
- Unprotected sex with more than one partner after another or without a change of condom

continued

Medium risk
- Vaginal or oral sex with a condom
- Giving oral sex to a man but not taking the ejaculate into the mouth
- Giving oral sex to a woman during her period but using a protection between yourself and the body fluids
- Giving oral sex to a woman but not during her period
- 'Rimming' with the protection of a barrier (e.g. dental dam*)
- 'Wet' kissing (French kissing) with open mouths depends on the health of your lips and mouth. Bleeding gums or ulcers, cut lips, cold sores, etc. increase the risk
- Sharing sex toys after washing (remove the batteries first) and covering with a fresh condom for each user
- Using a sex toy in the vagina after using it in the anus, with a fresh condom for each use

Low risk
- Masturbation on your own or with a partner (but make sure that any cuts or grazes are covered by a waterproof plaster or latex gloves)
- Use of personal sex toys (but make sure that they are washed after each use in warm soapy water)
- Kissing on the lips with no exchange of saliva or on the body
- Hugging, cuddling, body rubbing, sexual arousal fully clothed, licking food off each other or other activities that do not involve exchange of body fluids
- Sensual body massage (but ensure that oils do not come into contact with latex or rubber, which they can weaken)

continued

- Erotic fantasy, either alone or shared
- Anything else that gives mutual pleasure by mutual consent and that does not involve exchange of body fluids

*Dental dams are sheets of latex (rubber) used as a protection for oral sex. They should be placed over the whole of the area beforehand. They can fall off, so mark which side is yours or it defeats the object of protection if you replace it with the wrong side out! You can use a flavoured condom by splitting it up the long side to make a barrier.

Too much emphasis on the risks of STIs can be counter-productive. Young people often feel (perhaps rightly) that health professionals or other adults are making a mountain out of a molehill in order to control young people's sexuality. Straightforward factual information about the risks is all that is needed. Exaggeration or emotive language stops people listening. That is not to say that all the risks of sexual contact (including an unwanted pregnancy) should not be discussed, but they should be considered in the context of how enjoyable the activity can be as well!

Bear in mind that Peter Greenhouse[5] defined sexual health as the 'enjoyment of the sexual activity of one's choice without causing or experiencing physical or emotional harm'. Emphasising the downside of sexual activity can be just as harmful as receiving too little information to keep oneself safe.

References

1 Lamagni TL, Hughes G, Rogers PA, Paine T and Catchpole M (1999) New cases seen in genito-urinary medicine clinics: England 1998. *Comm Dis Rep Suppl.* **9**: S1–12.

2 Department of Health (1992) *The Health of the Nation.* HMSO, London.

3   Simms I, Catchpole M, Brugha R, Rogers P, Mallinson H and
    Nicoll A (1997) Epidemiology of genital *Chlamydia trachomatis*
    in England and Wales. *Genitourinary Med.* **73**: 122–6.

4   Hickson F, Weatherburn P, Reid D, Henderson L and
    Stephens M (1999) *Evidence for Change. Findings from the
    National Gay Men's Sex Survey.* Sigma Research, London.

5   Greenhouse P (1994) A sexual health service under one roof:
    setting up sexual health services for women. *J Matern Child
    Health.* **19**: 228–33.

► CHAPTER 11

Teenagers disadvantaged by disability or circumstances

Teenagers with learning disability

People with learning disability need to be able to access contraceptive and sexual health services, although their needs are often overlooked. Most people with learning disability need information and advice about their sexual development and appropriate behaviour as well as contraceptive care.

The *Health of the Nation* strategy[1] for people with learning disability recognised the increased risks of unwanted pregnancy if those with learning disability are less able to:

- understand the connection between sexual activity and pregnancy and sexually transmitted infections
- understand the responsibilities of parenthood
- assimilate information and advice about contraception and safer sex published in magazines
- receive or comprehend information given by peers about safer sex practices
- organise themselves to take regular contraception
- learn the skills of putting on a condom or inserting a cap at the appropriate time.

The *Health of the Nation* strategy emphasised the responsibilities of those providing education and care to teach people with learning disabilities about reproduction, contraception, making sexual choices and the responsibilities of parenthood.

As the majority of people with learning disability now live in the community rather than being isolated in mental hospitals, the bulk of their medical care is the responsibility of the primary healthcare and community learning disability teams. Many of those with learning disability have additional health problems, such as epilepsy, incontinence, sensory loss or behavioural problems. There has been widespread recognition that the health of those with learning disability may be neglected if health professionals do not take a proactive approach and undertake regular health checks to detect problems which may otherwise be neglected.[2,3] Advice about and help with sexual health and contraceptive matters might be offered routinely if general practices established annual health checks of people with learning disability organised through a practice database. Research to date has shown that general practitioners are reluctant to provide proactive health promotion for patients with learning disability,[4] and although adult patients with learning disability consult their general practitioners at equivalent rates to other patients, they receive less preventive care than do other patients. For instance, in a study of matched controls, individuals with learning disability were significantly less likely to have had a cervical smear in the previous five years.[5]

A total of 21 people with learning disability who were attending a local college were interviewed as part of a larger study auditing the effectiveness of contraceptive services for teenagers in the district. These students were aged 16 to 25 years, with a mean age of 18.8 years; 12 of them were females. Only one of the 21 students described herself as being sexually active. Most of the students were transported to and from the college by their parents and had few opportunities to socialise without supervision. Three of the students appeared to know about emergency contraception, and 18 students (86%) thought that they knew how to use a condom.[6]

Physical disability

People with profound physical disabilities also have problems with access to contraceptive and sexual health services. Just like those with learning disability, they may have few opportunities for sexual activities if they are isolated from their peers and closely supervised for most of the day. Able-bodied people such as health professionals, teachers and carers may overlook their needs and be unaware that people with significant physical disabilities are sexually active or would like to be, and therefore need advice and help with sexual and contraceptive matters.

Morgan Williams, who was Director of the Committee on Sexual Problems of the Disabled (SPOD) for 15 years, states that he:

'realised that the problems were usually with the carers and not the client group. The vast majority of disabled people were aware of what they could and could not do, who they wanted to do it with, when and where. The problems began for them when they needed to ask a carer for help, e.g. buying contraceptives, taking them to a social event, making an appointment, lifting them into bed with a partner or just affording them privacy. That often seemed to be the signal for the carer to project their own value system on to the situation and frequently say no, using risk as the reason.'[7]

J asked to see the doctor who worked with the disability team. He had talked to her before about masturbation, so knew that she would talk about sex with him. He wanted her to arrange for him and his newly found girlfriend to be able to meet somewhere other than the centre they both attended (when they were with lots of other people) and either of their homes. At his home, his mother left them

continued

> together in their wheelchairs, but kept popping in to 'see if they were all right'. Her mother stayed in the same room as them. He commented that she had obviously read his mind! The doctor found herself enquiring whether he had asked his girlfriend about sex. He put her nicely in her place by remarking 'Just because my legs don't work, it doesn't mean I can't use my mouth or my brain – and she's not daft either'.

Young people with physical disabilities need to be able to talk about their specific difficulties. Young people's disability teams often have someone available with a special interest and experience. Other health professionals can consult Cooper and Guillebaud's book,[7] *Sexuality and Disability*, for details of management in specific conditions.

Contraception needs to be tailored to the individual. Clear instructions are essential, especially if the teenager has visual, hearing or learning disabilities. Liaison with other medical advisers may be needed, especially if those advisers have little knowledge of contraception or have not thought about their patients' sexual needs.

Combined oral contraceptives (COCs)

Pill-taking is often complied with reliably by people with learning disability, and the COC may be a good choice because of the regular light periods that result from its use. Many people with learning disability have other medical problems. Phenobarbitone, phenytoin or carbamazepine are liver enzyme-inducing drugs, so higher doses of oestrogens should be given (50 mcg titrating to 90 mcg as combinations of standard pills).

Immobility in a wheelchair or localised movement loss (e.g. following cerebral palsy or spinal injury) increases the risk of thrombosis, so oestrogens should be avoided. COCs should also be avoided in people who have heart conditions that predispose to thrombosis. Some forms of Crohn's disease appear to worsen with oestrogens, so COCs should be avoided for them, too. Other conditions that cause diarrhoea can affect absorption, so avoid pills taken by mouth.

Progestogen-only pills (POPs)

POPs do not have the same thrombosis-promoting effect, so can be used by people with immobility. The irregular menstrual loss may be less well tolerated by people with learning disability. Remember that teenagers with diabetes may well be rebelling against the strict timing of their routine, so that this method – although very suitable in stable diabetics – may not be ideal during this particular phase of life. Interactions with enzyme-inducing drugs remain a problem, and the dose may need to be doubled or trebled. The dose should also be doubled in those who are very obese, as the failure rate appears to be increased if their weight exceeds 70 kg.

Progestogen injectables and implants

Although injection avoids the need for a good memory every day, some mechanism needs to be set up for arranging a follow-up appointment, as it is even easier to forget to return in 12 or 8 weeks for the next injection. Depo-Provera injections are particularly useful for those who wish to avoid or minimise menstrual loss, and are often used by women confined to wheelchairs or with learning disability. Weight gain can be a problem for those who are already at risk because of immobility. The light but irregular menstrual loss associated with Implanon implants may be less acceptable than that with Depo-Provera, but the lower progestogen dose is not likely to affect weight. Implanon only needs to be changed every three years, so may be useful for those who tend to forget to attend for injections.

> M was delighted when she experienced no menstrual bleeding at all after her second Depo-Provera injection. She had always found it very difficult to manage the hygiene necessary, as she wore adult nappies for her incontinence due to her spina bifida. Although she grumbled about having to control her weight more carefully (she was in a wheelchair and had little exercise), she went on to use this method for several years.

Intrauterine devices (IUD or IUS)

The main advantages of these devices are that no remembering is required – once fitted the device is always there ready – and they are highly effective. Copper-bearing devices tend to increase menstrual loss, which is a disadvantage if the woman is already having practical problems coping with the blood loss. A progestogen-bearing intrauterine system (Mirena) will reduce the loss, but irregular light loss will still occur, especially during the first 6–12 months.

Another disadvantage of the method is the practical difficulty of inserting an IUD when physical disability makes positioning with the legs apart problematic. The position used for intercourse may be the best one to use for IUD insertion, so the inserter needs to be expert and willing to work in awkward positions. Someone with learning difficulty or with athetosis may have problems keeping still enough. Insertion of an IUD through the cervix in someone with a spinal injury may cause automatic dysreflexia with a sharp rise in blood pressure, and should only be undertaken with ready access to emergency medical treatment.

Careful counselling is needed to ensure that women with learning disability understand fully what is going to be done and why. The use of a general anaesthetic is no substitute for full understanding. Local anaesthesia is a sensible adjunct to a comfortable fitting, but if a thorough understanding is obtained, then follow-up and changing the IUD will not be distressing.

Barrier methods (diaphragm or cap, male or female condoms)

Putting in a diaphragm that has been made slippery with spermicide can be a challenge to fully able-bodied women, let alone those in whom physical disability impairs mobility or dexterity. Involving the partner can be an advantage, as can shared responsibility for putting on a condom – four handicapped hands can substitute for two fully functional ones. Remember that people with learning disability tend to take teaching very literally, so be very clear about where the diaphragm or condom is to be fitted. The use of a model may be confusing and lead to incorrect use. Advice about emergency contraception should always accompany instruction about barrier methods.

Sterilisation

This is not a method of choice for any young person, whatever their problems or parental concerns. Situations change and medical advances occur, but sterilisation should be regarded as irreversible. A long-acting method such as the progestogen-bearing intrauterine system (Mirena) or an implant like Implanon gives time for change to occur and enables the situation to be reconsidered at intervals.

Teenagers in care

Less than 1% of each age group is brought up 'in care' through foster care or in children's homes, but those leaving care are over-represented among the homeless, the unemployed, teenage single parents and the prison population.[8]

Those in care often come from deprived social and economic backgrounds. They are more likely to come from homes with a single parent or from overcrowded accommodation.[9] While in care they are often moved from one home to another, and truancy and educational neglect are common. The vast majority of young people leaving care have received a poor education and have few qualifications. Most of them leave care at 16 years of age to compete with everyone else for housing and jobs. In one study, nearly half of the teenagers had become parents within two years of leaving care.[10] Young homeless teenagers are vulnerable to drug abuse, crime, violence, sexual abuse and prostitution.

Better provision of both contraception and healthcare advice and services both while in care and immediately afterwards could have a significant impact on the misery and destitution of many of these young people. Healthcare workers need to unite with Social Services and 'floating support schemes' and hostels for the homeless to provide better access to contraception and healthcare. Local authorities are required to prepare young people for leaving care, and can support them up to the age of 21 years, but care-leaving schemes are underresourced and patchy.

Drug users, prostitutes and prisoners

Most drug users are young and frequently change sexual partners. People who inject drugs are particularly likely to acquire HIV by that route and then risk spreading the virus by sexual contact (*see* Chapter 10 on sexually transmitted illnesses for advice on safer sex). A sizeable proportion of male drug users have non-drug using female partners. A significant number of drug users occasionally work as prostitutes.[11] Within the UK, reports of positive HIV tests are growing fastest among those believed to be infected through heterosexual contact, but there is a failure to recognise that homosexual contact is not the only risk. A study in London found that heroin smokers who had not injected had a 3.6% HIV infection rate[11] from hetero-sexual intercourse.

Drugs lower inhibitions, and many young people report that they had unprotected intercourse while under the influence of alcohol or cannabis. Emergency contraception and infection screening should follow exposure. Everyone needs to have a greater awareness of the risks. Teenagers with higher self-esteem and more self-assertiveness can say 'No' to too much alcohol, illegal drugs *and* unwanted intercourse.

One study of drug injectors in England estimated that 7–10% of them had accepted money or drugs for sex. The majority of professional prostitutes of either sex know the risks, and the levels of HIV infection among female prostitutes are low. In Glasgow, all of the female prostitutes who were found to be HIV-positive (2.3%) were also drug injectors.[11] Drug users or professional sex workers should take appro-priate precautions (e.g. use stronger condoms). Male prosti-tutes are often at a disadvantage. They are usually paid after the transaction, and the client usually makes the decision about whether a condom is worn. Female prostitutes are often adept at applying condoms in an arousing way, and either refuse a client or charge them much higher fees for sex without a condom, as a deterrent. Those who are most at risk are the drug users or homeless people who 'sell' sex in exchange for drugs, food or shelter.

A large number of drug users will spend some of their time in prison. Many homeless people or those who have been in care will also spend time in prison. Drug use may occur for the first time in prison or the type of use may change. Homosexual sexual encounters are common in prisons, but condoms are usually only issued for use on home visits. The lack of acknowledgement of sexual behaviour in prison leads to a lack of protection. Those who inject drugs in prison are very likely to share equipment, and the risk of HIV infection is increased. After discharge many people are left homeless and living on the street with increased risks of unprotected inter-course. Numerous publications have advocated pre-release planning and support after discharge, but even where this is available, suspicion of those in authority and alienation from cultural norms often prevent uptake of the service.

References

1   Department of Health (1995) *A Strategy for People with Learning Disabilities. The Health of the Nation*. Department of Health, London.

2   Lindsey M and Russell O (1999) *Once a Day*. NHS Executive, London.

3   Martin G and Lindsey M (1999) People with learning disabilities in the community: where do we go from here? *Br J Gen Pract*. **49**: 751 (letter).

4   Kerr M, Dunstan F and Thapar A (1996) Attitudes of general practitioners to caring for people with learning disability. *Br J Gen Pract*. **46**: 92–4.

5   Whitfield M, Langar J and Russell O (1995) Assessing general practitioners' care of adult patients with learning disability: case–control study. *Qual Health Care*. **5**: 31–5.

6   Chambers R and Milsom G (1997) Knowledge of contraception and sexual experiences of young people with learning disabilities. *SLD Exp: Br Inst Learn Disabil*. **17**: 9–10.

7   Williams M (1999) Foreword. In: E Cooper and J Guillebaud (eds) *Sexuality and Disability*. Radcliffe Medical Press, Oxford.

8   Anderson L, Kemp P and Quilgars D (1993) *Single Homeless People*. HMSO, London.

9   Bebbington A and Miles J (1989) The background of children who enter local authority care. *Br J Soc Work*. **19**: 349–68.

10 Biehal N, Clayden J, Stein M and Wade J (1995) *Moving On: young people and leaving care schemes*. HMSO, London.

11 Department of Health (1993) *AIDS and Drug Misuse Update*. HMSO, London.

CHAPTER 12

Culture, religion and beliefs

Sexuality and contraception are private and personal parts of our lives, but religion and the State have always been involved in trying to exercise control over them. Sexuality is a matter of both private and public concern, and the way in which it should be conducted is learned through interactions at home and at school, through the media and, for many, through religious teachings.

Healthcare workers are conscious of the difficulties they face when in contact with people who have different belief systems or cultural and religious backgrounds. They fear that they will give offence by not knowing what those beliefs are, and they often make attempts to find out some general information that will help them or make them feel that they are more in control of the situation. Unfortunately, this tendency for health professionals to want to be in control, or to be seen as having a superior level of knowledge, can cause them difficulties. Lists of cultural norms are of limited usefulness, and may be applied in rigid and potentially discriminatory ways.[1] Each person's interpretation of his or her culture will be different, and there are as many differences within each cultural system as there are between cultures. It is essential to establish what it means for that person – not to be 'in control' but to acknowledge the greater knowledge of that individual about what he or she believes.

Attitudes and beliefs that are held publicly sometimes bear little resemblance to what is practised in private relationships.

Beliefs and values may have to be modified by circumstances, and this can cause real distress if there is a conflict between the two. Others modify the strictures of their faith or culture without apparently experiencing any distress.

The complex interaction between different sets of values or standards can sometimes lead to conflicts with health professionals, who are unable to understand the reasons behind what appear to them to be irrational decisions or behaviour.

> The woman in Asian dress who attends to have her intrauterine device removed and then reattends a few months later for its reinsertion, can seem silly and irritating to the doctor, especially if she is reluctant to explain the real reasons for her requests because she is afraid she will not be understood. In fact, she may have changed to the progestogen injection just while she was travelling on a pilgrimage, as it would be important that she did not bleed during this time.
>
> A Western girl who wishes to do the same while travelling the world during her year off before going to university would feel able to explain her reasons without fear of disapproval, because she would assume that she and the doctor share the same cultural values. However, it is just as misguided to assume that people who share the same cultural background have similar ideas. The doctor may well disapprove of young women who travel abroad in this way, perhaps because the doctor was not able to do so when she or he was young and is therefore envious of the girl or perhaps because a daughter of his or hers ran into trouble while travelling in this way.

Gender and sexuality

Sexuality is both biologically driven and subject to social construction and modification. It is clear from historical and anthropological studies that sexual identity and practices have varied according to both time and geographical location.

For young men passing through adolescence today, sexual issues seem to be focused around access and prowess. They often perceive the formation of their identity of manhood or masculinity in terms of their sexual activity. Promiscuous boys are often praised or at least receive tacit approval. For young women, sexuality is viewed as a much more risky business, and girls who behave in a similar way to many boys are vilified as deserving all that happens to them (pregnancy or disease) as a punishment.

In the Western world, ideas about sexuality have been constructed around the stereotypes of the madonna and the whore for many years. Women have been regarded either as pure, innocent and chaste or as voracious sexual harlots. Women who were sexually active have been condemned, especially if they were active in this way outside marriage. Although attitudes have moderated to some extent over time, anyone who has listened to a rape trial will know how much emphasis is placed on the previous sexual activity of the victim, as if being sexually experienced somehow made her less deserving of respect. Many women have complained that they feel as if they are on trial as much as the rapist.

Women have been discriminated against on account of their sexual activity for many years. In recent history women were placed in psychiatric hospitals because they were unmarried and pregnant. Some of them remained in long-term care because they had nowhere else to go after such disgrace had befallen them. Prostitutes were (and still are) blamed for their work and for being the source of sexually transmitted illnesses. In the UK, the Contagious Diseases Acts from 1864 to 1883 were directed against women working as prostitutes. The language used was moralistic and accusatory. In contrast, the examination of soldiers for STIs was abandoned in 1859 because it was considered repugnant to the feelings of men.[2]

Even today, women sex workers are regarded as sources of HIV infection of heterosexual men, rather than as being more at risk from their clients because of the greater likelihood of transmission of HIV from males to females.[3] They still suffer disproportionate prosecution for soliciting, compared to the rarer prosecutions of their clients. The women are blamed for being available, rather than the men being blamed for being unable to control their sexual appetites or desires.

If one believes that sexuality is only acceptable if one is male, then young women believe that if they carry condoms they will be branded as sluts.[4] Young women often know about safe sex, and intend to use condoms, but find themselves unable to be assertive enough to do this within the context of a sexual relationship. They feel that they should be passive and undemanding, and that the man should take the lead.

Young men are confused, too. How can they take the lead with these apparently more confident and knowledgeable young women? Whatever they do will be wrong. If they do not pressurise for sex early in the relationship, they fear that they will be branded as wimps. However, if they try for sex too early, they may well be accused of only wanting women for sex. They are encouraged to despise the 'easy' sexual conquest (as 'cheap' and having no value), but equally they brand women who resist their sexual advances as 'frigid'. How can they ever get it right?

Despite this, women are frequently viewed as being responsible for controlling men's sexual urges as well as their own. Men's irresponsible behaviour is condoned as natural, and this attitude has a major impact on teenage pregnancy rates and sexually transmitted illnesses.

Some feminists have promoted the idea that the concept and practice of sexuality are inherently masculine or are designed to increase the power of men over women. They have proposed that vaginal penetration should be avoided or that withdrawal (i.e. men controlling their sexuality to protect against pregnancy) should be the method of choice. Some feminists have proposed that the oral contraceptive pill, far from liberating women, has encouraged men to behave even more recklessly and to use women as a source of free access for male pleasure.

There are real difficulties involved in reconciling women's sexuality as a source of pleasure and the reality that expression of their sexuality exposes them to risk. Anxiety about the availability of contraception raises the issue of whether sexual enjoyment is legitimate for young teenagers under the (state-imposed) age of consent. During the early eighteenth century the age of consent was 12 years for young women and 14 years for young men. Early marriage and lack of contraception produced equally early pregnancies and high mortality and morbidity rates among both young mothers and infants. The gradual lengthening of the time of dependency of adolescents upon their parents has decreased their autonomy and at the same time incorporated a denial of their sexuality.

Young people are not only inexperienced in life but are also financially dependent either on their parents or on state provision (where this is available). Young men cannot look forward with confidence to a separate existence in employment, and their traditional role models (if present) are also likely to suffer from periods of unemployment and loss of power and identity within the family environment.

Regretted sexual intercourse

Several studies have indicated that sexual intercourse before the age of 16 years is often regretted. Two of these studies[5,6] were based on recall of what people did several years previously, and might have been biased by a re-evaluation of earlier behaviour as immature or inconsiderate.

However, a more recent study of representative 14-year-olds in Scotland[7] confirmed the earlier findings. It found that 18% of boys and 15% of girls reported that they had had heterosexual intercourse since their thirteenth birthday. Around 40% of them thought that intercourse had happened at about the right time, while 27% of the boys and 32% of the girls reported that it had happened too early. Reports of being pressured, exerting pressure, not having planned intercourse and relatively high levels of parental monitoring were all significantly associated with regret.

Anticipated regret about sexual intercourse is associated with a higher degree of planning (and contraceptive use[8]). Spreading the word that many teenagers regret exerting pressure and not planning their first intercourse might help other young people to postpone instant gratification in favour of later satisfaction.

Youth cultures

Closer examination of youth cultures reveals a wide disparity. Some individuals may already be parents, while others are still emotionally child-like. Some may have travelled widely, while others have never left their home environment. They may be students, employed or unemployed, but many of them are not financially independent. Differences in class, ethnicity, sexual orientation, religious beliefs or lack of them, education and expectations make them a diverse group, with shared youthfulness being the only common denominator.

'Adults' – that is, older people – frequently find young people threatening, particularly when they hang around in groups, because they do not understand their belief systems. Young people may appear to be alien beings who do not conform to the standards expected and are often castigated for believing in nothing at all. Any investigation into what young people do believe in is inevitably out of date by the time it is completed, but it can give some insight and common ground from which to explore what 'life' means for an individual.

Stainton Rogers and colleagues[9] describe three value patterns that were obtained by giving lists of values to focus groups of young people and asking them to rate them according to their importance. They identified several common themes, which are described below.

Hedonistic companionship

The value that was rated highest was happiness, with the major route to happiness being warm and close relationships with friends and family. This bears similarities to the Acid House culture of the 1980s, with its search for pleasure in dance and music (and sometimes drug use) and a secret separate youth identity of its members' own choosing.

Streetwise individualism

The 'wisdom' valued so highly was described in the focus group discussions as a kind of worldly-wise cynicism. Crucial to this wisdom was the ability not to be conned. Young people wished to be able to trust their own judgement and not be swayed by politicians or advertising. They valued their ability to 'do their own thing,' and they distrusted institutions and authority.

Born-again salvation

Young people who had strong religious beliefs or affiliations put a comfortable life or social recognition very low on their scale of values, with 'salvation' rated as being most important.

The characteristics that the group members valued the most were being a responsible companion, being a fun-loving companion or being a 'mover and shaker'.

> A responsible companion was identified as follows: 'what matters is to be somebody that your friends can rely on'.
>
> The fun-loving companion was identified as follows: 'the kind of person who's great to be with, good fun' or as 'it's about being connected, the incredible feeling you get of being part of something bigger'.
>
> A mover and shaker was identified as someone who knows where they are going and has the intelligence, energy and ambition to go far: 'you need to have a dream, to settle on what you want and go for it'.[9]

The young people in the focus groups had quite traditional hopes for the future. They wanted a comfortable lifestyle, a home of their own, a car and a reasonably satisfying and well-paid job. Most of them envisaged themselves settling down and having children, but they saw this as a long-term goal, and expressed concerns that it would be more difficult for them to achieve than it had been for their parents. They were particularly concerned that they could not see themselves being able to do worthwhile jobs, and many of them spoke of 'opting out of the rat race' and settling for short-term, insecure jobs interspersed with periods on welfare benefits. In contrast, some of them were extremely ambitious and determined to become rich and famous, and they were willing to work hard and make sacrifices to get there.

These 'snapshots' of what groups of young people in 1994 thought about their own standards and beliefs contradict adult perceptions that young people have no values. They also demonstrate the diversity of belief systems, and reinforce the need to treat each person as an individual with his or her own values and aspirations. Without some understanding of that belief system, trying to negotiate a plan for the future (e.g. post-ponement of pleasure for future gain or contraception rather than conception) is doomed to failure.

The 'underclass' or 'subculture'

The media frequently describe sections of the population who do not conform to everyday stereotypes in these terms. These vulnerable individuals find it difficult to gain access to any kind of help, being socially deprived and often struggling to exist in inner cities or isolated in rural communities. They are often suspicious of authority and fear loss of confidentiality if anyone knows their business (especially if it is not legal). They fear professional scorn and often view what happens to them fatalistically. They do not feel that they have any control over their own lives, and if pregnancy occurs they believe that it is due to fate.

They regard contraception as the imposition of yet another control by others over their own lives, and they often go to ridiculous lengths to circumvent the efforts that are made 'on their behalf'.

> They are out when the domiciliary family planning health professional calls, they cannot remember when the clinic or surgery is open, they forget their pills or the timing of the next injection, and they even remove their own intrauterine devices.

Sexual activity is free and enjoyable, and making babies may be the only skill that they have. Having babies to care for can compensate for unemployment, lack of fulfilment and poor self-esteem.

It is important to beware of making judgements in these circumstances. Some of the teenagers who are caught in this

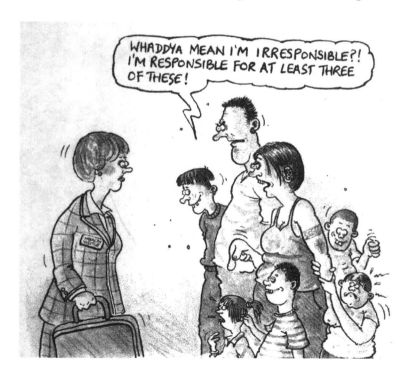

trap are transformed after maternity into strong-willed people who decide to break out of their poverty by obtaining qualifications and training for 'proper' jobs, despite the manifest mountains they have to climb in order to do so. Others join the cycle of deprivation in which all the women from each generation have babies at an early age, are unmarried, and have several successive partners who fail to support them in any way.

Travellers or Romanies

Despite often appearing to fit into the above category, the extended family structure and support in these groups gives them a different identity and resilience. Women are often also financially supported by a partner. If they have no stable site from which they travel out, they may have difficulty accessing health services and their health may suffer as a result. Their education is also affected, and many have a poor knowledge of their bodies and are insufficiently literate to read explanatory leaflets about contraception. They sometimes also have a poor grasp of appointment systems or times.

> An attractive 17-year-old girl attended a Friday evening surgery. She found it difficult to express herself clearly, but with increasing irritation the doctor discovered that this patient had registered with the practice just prior to the birth of her now 4-week-old infant. She wanted a coil fitted tonight – now. She could not return next week, as they would be 'on their way' tomorrow.

Beware of making assumptions – some travellers are highly self-educated and articulate! Health professionals need to consider how to adapt their contraceptive and sexual health advice to meet the needs of these people, especially if they will be travelling to another area before long. Methods of contraception that require regular attendance (e.g. progestogen injections or supplies of pills) may not be feasible. Intrauterine devices seem to be popular, despite the disadvantages of having to cope with heavier periods in a caravan or bus. A diaphragm seems to appeal to some travellers as it is a method that does not involve issues of authority, unlike other methods!

African-Caribbean communities

Many of the original immigrant communities have lived in the UK for several generations, and cultural changes have occurred during this time, tending to polarise the community. Some are extremely wary of white professionals, who they suspect are trying to control their fertility, while others have embraced religion, chastity or strict family controls.

Many families exist as matriarchal communities. Birth outside marriage does not carry a stigma, and proof of fertility is highly regarded. Evidence of regular menstruation is often regarded as important, and consequently injectable progestogens are usually unpopular. Some members of this group may have sickle-cell anaemia, and Depo-Provera has beneficial effects in preventing crises in this condition.

Many African-Caribbeans have a slow acetylator status, which means that they metabolise drugs more slowly. Complaints about intolerance of COCs may possibly be due to this effect, and a lower-dose pill should be suggested. African-Caribbeans are also more susceptible to hypertension, and this could be exacerbated by oestrogen-containing contraceptives.

Rastafarians

Contraception is unacceptable to most Rastafarians, and is regarded as an attempt on the part of white society to control black fertility. 'Natural' methods may sometimes be acceptable. A few Rastafarians appear to use their religion to justify irresponsible sexual behaviour with its increased risk of sexually transmitted diseases. Many Rastafarians in the UK see the movement as a paramilitary organisation rather than a religion.

Bah'i faith

This religion originated in Persia in the nineteenth century and emphasises the harmony of science and religion and the equality of men and women.[10] The bearing of children is a prime consideration in marriage, but the use of contraception is left to the conscience of the individual couple. Many who practise this faith prefer not to use methods of contraception that may work by preventing the implantation of a fertilised egg. Offers of intrauterine devices need to include information about the reduction in fertilisation that occurs with copper-bearing devices, and post-coital methods may be unacceptable.

Buddhism

Buddhists are enjoined to undertake to avoid intentional harm to any living (i.e. breathing) thing. Contraception is not usually a problem, as harm cannot be done to a non-existent being. However, Buddhism is very open to individual interpretation and definitions of existence may vary between different cultures and belief systems. It is important to explore individual beliefs during counselling about contraception (as should indeed be done with everyone).

Chinese

Many cities in the UK have Chinese communities. They tend to live in small groups close together, as many of them arrived as refugees and felt alone and isolated from their family members. Almost all Chinese are Buddhists. The close-knit nature of the community can cause problems for relationships that develop with outsiders. There is often little opportunity for young people to be alone together – an effective contraceptive in itself – and their high aspirations for further education and training also tend to postpone sexual activity until later.

Vietnamese

Many Vietnamese also arrived in the UK as refugees, and large families have been traditionally regarded with pride. Young Vietnamese people often have limited knowledge of contraception, and sex education is viewed with some suspicion. Religious persecution by the Vietnamese State has made them wary about discussing their religious beliefs in response to questions from individuals they regard as authority figures (e.g. doctors). Some young people may be Buddhists or Taoists, but many Vietnamese in the UK are Catholics.

Catholicism

The Catholic Church teaches that the vocation of love can only be fulfilled in two ways:

- through marriage characterised by faithfulness, permanence and openness to life
- through virginity or chastity.

The teaching about contraception refers only to that within marriage, as the question of contraception outside marriage does not arise. Natural methods are the only permitted ones, and specialised instruction is available from most family planning services or from the Catholic Marriage Advisory Council.

According to fertility studies,[11] all methods of contraception are used in practice, and some priests will advise women or couples to use their own conscience to weigh up the risks and benefits of childbearing. The oral contraceptive is sometimes prescribed as a menstruation regulator, and intercourse recommended for 'mid-cycle'. However, some Catholic women will be distressed and uncomfortable about using contraception because of their religious beliefs, and will probably chop and change, as no method will ever be entirely satisfactory.

Christian Science

Christian Scientists are free to make their own decisions with regard to family planning. However, they prefer to be free of drugs and all forms of medication, including hormonal contraception. Freedom from sexual activity is promoted as an aid to spirituality.

Church of England

Contraception is usually acceptable without any constraints. However, sexual activity outside marriage is not acceptable, and conflicts may arise between family members during adolescence, with rebellion of young people against parental standards.

Church of Jesus Christ of the Latter-day Saints (Mormons)

Procreation is encouraged and sterilisation is only permitted after permission has been granted by a bishop. Family responsibilities are taken very seriously, and strict constraints and controls restrict adolescent behaviour.

Hinduism

Hindus are primarily in favour of reproduction, and many of them believe that it is their duty to produce a son, since only sons can perform the funeral rites that enable a man's soul to go to heaven. Contraception is generally only practised after the birth of a son. Partial abstinence from sex is expected, especially during some religious festivals. Abortion is prohibited unless the mother's life is in danger.

A wide range of attitudes towards contraception exists among Hindus in the UK, ranging from the views of traditionalists, who would never consider any form of contraception, to more westernised ideas about control of fertility and the quality of life. The diaphragm is not a good method, as most Hindus believe that the right hand should not touch the genitals. Women may find genital examination distressing, as they should only be touched by their husbands. They may refuse to be examined by a male health professional, and some will wish to cover their faces during internal examinations. The intrauterine device may not be chosen for this reason or because it can prolong periods, as Hindu women cannot attend prayers or perform certain household tasks while they are menstruating.

The most popular method is the condom, but many women will now take the contraceptive pill. Many Hindus are vegetarian and may therefore need to know whether the pills contain animal products.

Recently arrived immigrants tend to have a limited general knowledge of contraception, and Hindus vary widely in their customs and beliefs. Adolescents growing up in the UK face conflicts between their traditional culture and that of the world around them. Arranged marriages and expectations of chastity before marriage are common, and sexual activity before marriage or with someone from another religion or culture may cause much distress and heart-searching.

Islam

Premarital sex is prohibited. Contraception is permitted in order to space childbearing to promote the health of an existing child or if there is concern about the physical or mental well-being of the mother. Withdrawal is permitted, and most Muslims will allow other non-permanent methods, such as barrier methods, hormonal contraceptives or intrauterine devices. Abortion is forbidden, as is vasectomy. Some conservative Muslims regard contraception as interfering with God's design.

Infertility can have serious consequences and may even result in rejection and divorce. Beliefs about women's roles and responsibilities influence parental decisions about the education and upbringing of their daughters in the UK, and these girls and young women are often segregated away from non-Muslims. Marriage is compulsory for both sexes, and women are under the guardianship of a man – the father, husband or (if widowed) sons. Some women come into conflict with health professionals who do not understand that permission must be obtained from the husband before any decision about the contraceptive method can be made.

Any method of contraception that prolongs or causes irregular periods may be unacceptable, as Muslim women who are menstruating cannot fast during Ramadan or visit the mosque. They may refuse examination within 10 days of their period, and insertion of an intrauterine device may be refused during or immediately after menstruation, which causes some difficulties in establishing the absence of pregnancy before fitting the device. Touching the genitals with the right hand is prohibited, and this makes diaphragm fitting difficult.

Jehovah's Witnesses

Contraception is considered to be a matter of personal conscience, but abortion or methods that work by preventing implantation of a fertilised egg are incompatible with their religious beliefs. Family values are important, and extramarital or premarital sexual activity is unacceptable.

Judaism

Sources in Jewish law state that a man cannot use any form of contraception. However, as women are not mentioned, most interpret this as meaning that women may do so. Hormonal methods are acceptable for those who believe that 'no physical impediment' may be used, as no male sperm are destroyed or prevented from ingress. Even the strictly religious may seek permission from the Rabbi to space their children in order to preserve health, although the edict to 'go forth and multiply' is often taken seriously. Marriages are often arranged and extramarital or premarital sexual activity is forbidden. In very orthodox circles the sexes are segregated from about 7–8 years of age, but most Jews live more relaxed social lives and interpret their religion on a more individual basis.

Women may not attend the temple or have intercourse during menstruation and for seven days afterwards (when a bath ritual is performed). Methods that prolong menstruation or cause more frequent blood loss are unpopular. Abortion is not permitted unless the mother's life is at risk or occasionally if a congenital disease is detected in early pregnancy.

Sikhs

Sikh women are highly respected and have a large influence in domestic and community matters. High moral character, modesty and sexual morality are very important, and sexual activity outside marriage is not expected to occur. It is important for couples to have a son, but otherwise contraception is welcomed and the family size is usually limited. Sikh women often select their own method of contraception without encountering opposition from their husbands, and are often seen to be independent and authoritative.[12]

Female genital mutilation

Female genital mutilation is widely practised and accepted in many African countries and in some parts of the Middle East and Asia.[13] It may involve cutting off the hood of the clitoris (which is known as excision of the clitoris) with or without removal of the labia minora. Infibulation, which is the most drastic procedure, involves removal of the clitoris, the labia minora and most of the labia majora. The remnants are then sewn together to provide a small passageway for urine and menstrual flow. Women may ask for help with problems of non-consummation, infertility, painful periods, vaginal or urinary tract infections and psychosexual problems.

Conclusion

The above is not intended to be a definitive list of all the various cultural or religious influences you may encounter, but it does provide some clues as to why couples or individuals may have difficulty in establishing a rapport with health professionals. Not all of the people who appear to have the same cultural or religious background will behave (or believe) in the same way, and some second- or third-generation immigrants will have modified their belief systems to a greater or lesser extent.

Popular literature nearly always assumes that teenagers are heterosexual and sexually active. For some people the results of sexual activity outside marriage are disgrace and shame on all the family. The exploration of relationship forming and emphasis on sexual activity can totally exclude many young people of Asian origin. Similarly, teenage homosexual relationships are actively discouraged or ignored. The peer group pressure to conform to a heterosexual 'norm' alienates those who are not so inclined, and can cause much distress.

It is important to be aware that religion and culture can have profound influences both on behaviour and on the way that women and men feel about their sexuality. Make sure that you understand your own belief systems so that you do not unwittingly try to impose them on others inappropriately. Enquire sensitively about people's belief systems and backgrounds in order to help them to make sense of their sexual activities and needs, and always tailor your advice on sexual activity and contraception to the needs of the individual.

References

1   Montford H and Skrine R (eds) (1993) *Contraceptive Care: meeting individual needs*. Chapman & Hall, London.

2   Davenport-Hines R (1990) *Sex, Death and Punishment*. Fontana, London.

3   Johnston M and Johnstone F (1993) *HIV Infections in Women*. Churchill Livingstone, Edinburgh.

4   Holland J, Ramazanoglu C and Scott S (1990) *Women, Risk and AIDS. Project Papers 1–8*. Tufnell Press, London.

5   Johnson AM, Wadsworth J, Wellings K and Field J (1994) *Sexual Attitudes and Lifestyles*. Blackwell Scientific Publications, Oxford.

6   Dickson N, Paul C, Herbison P and Silva P (1998) First sexual intercourse: age, coercion and later regrets. *BMJ*. **316**: 29–33.

7   Wight D, Henderson M, Raab G *et al.* (2000) Extent of regretted sexual intercourse among young teenagers in Scotland: a cross-sectional survey. *BMJ*. **320**: 1243–4.

8   Richard R, van der Pligt J and de Vries NK (1996) Anticipated regret and time perspective: changing sexual risk-taking behaviour. *J Behav Decision Making*. **3**: 262–77.

9   Stainton Rogers W, Stainton Rogers R, Výrost J and Lovás L (1997) Worlds apart: young people's aspirations in a changing Europe. In: J Roche & S Tucker (eds) *Youth in Society*. Sage Publications, London.

10 Contraceptive Education Service (2000) *Religion and Contraception, Factsheet No 15*. Family Planning Association, London.

11 Cartwright A (1976) *How Many Children?* Routledge & Kegan Paul, London.

12 Leicester City Council (1986) *Religious Background of Asians in Leicester City Survey*. Leicester City Council, Leicester.

13 Ng F (2000) Female genital mutilation: its implications for reproductive health. An overview. *Br J Fam Plan*. **26**: 47–51.

► CHAPTER 13

Abuse and teenagers

Introduction

The younger the teenager who presents to a health professional, the more care has to be taken to ensure that the patient understands the consequences of their actions. It is particularly important to be aware of the possibility that the young person is the victim of abuse or exploitation. Healthcare workers need to be aware of the local child abuse guidelines and procedures and to be able to refer to them if suspicions are raised. The Social Services department has a legal duty to 'make available such advice, guidance and assistance as may promote the welfare of children by diminishing the need to receive children into or keep them in care'. Social Services can receive a child into care on a voluntary basis if the parents are unable to care for their child and care by relatives or others cannot be arranged.

Healthcare workers need to know that they can approach Social Services, the police or the National Society for the Prevention of Cruelty to Children (NSPCC), or other specific individuals such as the responsible paediatrician, for an investigation if abuse is either suspected or complained of by a child. Mutually supportive contact between local families, voluntary groups and neighbourhood projects has a role to play in each community.

A child or young person who appears to be abused or neglected can be removed to a place of safety for 28 days on application to a magistrate. The Social Services department or the NSPCC normally do this, and action should be taken in conjunction with the Social Services department. The police can detain a child in a 'place of safety' for up to 8 days while seeking the aid of Social Services for care proceedings. Sometimes there is a dilemma as to how much action a health professional should initiate, especially when standards of care are very different to what the health professional considers to be satisfactory.

The welfare of the child or young person is of paramount concern, and the gathering of evidence about the abuse should not become an additional source of abuse. Avoid repeated interviewing or examination by rapidly referring abused young people to individuals with special expertise and training. Healthcare workers and others who have long-term involvement with abused young people require regular supervision and support. Work in this area makes considerable emotional demands, and there is a tendency to over-identify with a particular individual within the family and become drawn into collusive behaviour if one has not received proper training and support.

Child abuse

Verbal or emotional abuse may occur if parents or guardians continually fail to show their children love and affection. They may shout at the children, only notice them when they do things wrong or threaten them with retribution or abandonment.

Bruising, cuts, burns, fractures or other injuries are signs of physical abuse. Physical neglect occurs if children are not protected from danger or are inadequately fed, clothed or kept warm.

A 13- or 14-year-old out on the streets of a town or city in the dark, unfed except for a bag of chips, wearing thin

continued

clothing that gives poor protection from the weather, and who is unable or too fearful to return home is at risk of exploitation or criminal activity.

Young people may self-harm or behave in a risky way due to feelings of worthlessness and low self-esteem. Abused children lack self-esteem, become bullies or withdrawn and isolated, and often seek emotional reward outside the home. They may want to have a baby who will love them (they think) or seek out inappropriate sexual relationships because they have no idea of how to relate to other people in any other way. They are vulnerable to exploitation by others because of their low self-worth.

Young women often believe that they will not have a boyfriend unless they consent to sex, at the same time believing that if they do have sex they will be thought of as having little value. No wonder they are confused. Young men often believe that they must have sex in order to conceal how inadequate and weak they feel. They regard sex as a weapon to demonstrate their power. These young men and women do not dare to show their feelings, and instead conceal them behind bravado and antisocial behaviour.

Sexual abuse

A useful definition of sexual abuse has been provided by Kempe and Kempe:[1]

'The involvement of dependent, developmentally immature children and adolescents in sexual activities which they do not truly comprehend and to which they are unable to give informed consent, or which violate the taboos of family roles'.

The sexual exploitation of teenagers may be a continuation of earlier abuse that has been occurring since they were much younger or it may first start in adolescence. It can vary from genital fondling to oral, vaginal or anal penetration. The exploitation involves an imbalance of power[2] between the abuser and their victim because of age difference, authority or threat.

Sexual abuse occurs mainly within families by relatives. It may occur outside the family by someone known to the victim, and is occasionally perpetrated by strangers. Much of the abuse is by parents, and it is more common in families where the male perpetrator is not the biological father. Sexual abuse is more commonly reported in females, but it is extremely difficult for boys or men to admit to having experienced abusive episodes, and the numbers recorded may be an underestimate of the real situation.[3] Children have sexual feelings from a very young age, but sexuality in childhood should be different to that in adult life. If sexual abuse occurs, the boundaries between adult and child have become confused and the trust of the dependent child is betrayed. Children may co-operate, agree to activities and sometimes enjoy them, but they cannot give free, informed consent. The misuse of power may include sexual activities in the context of warmth and love, the granting of a special status or privileges, bribery or extreme secrecy.

Effects of abuse

Abuse is not a uniform problem. It may vary from a single episode of indecent exposure or genital fondling to systematic penetrative activities by a male over many years. Sexual abuse that is accompanied by emotional and/or physical abuse may be more damaging than sexual abuse in a loving (albeit abnormal) relationship between parent and child. The way in which people are supported when they disclose the abuse will also affect the extent of their later symptoms.

The long-term effects of abuse have mainly been described in patients who are psychiatrically disturbed. They range from no apparent effects to failure to form lasting emotional relationships, and sexual coldness. Promiscuity is described, often associated with alcohol or other drug misuse. Those who have been abused have a low sense of self-worth, they are often depressed and may describe a sense of contamination or dirtiness.

Tsai and colleagues[4] compared girls who felt damaged by their experiences with a matched group who did not. Those who were affected tended to have had more frequent abuse over a longer duration, with penetration being more likely. Those who were unaffected tended to have had more support from family and friends during childhood, and had not been blamed for the events. They also tended to have more supportive relationships in adult life.

Edwards and Donaldson[5] used a self-reporting questionnaire to assess the range of commonly reported symptoms in adult survivors of incest. They identified typical stress responses that were identical to those experienced by survivors of other traumatic events. Vulnerability and isolation, fear and anxiety, anger and feelings of betrayal, sadness and feelings of loss were usual. Shame, guilt and powerlessness accompanied avoidance of activities that provoked memories of the abuse. A general lack of responsiveness to the outside world produced a type of defence against feeling.

Adolescents may 'act out' in a dramatic fashion by becoming involved with drugs, by self-harm or suicide attempts, becoming out of control of their parents or school or running away from home. Associations have been described between a history of previous sexual abuse and teenage pregnancy,[6] anorexia nervosa and teenage prostitution.[7] Both failure at school and paradoxical over-achievement may result from childhood abuse.

Identification of abuse

Abuse is common, and suspicions that a teenager may be being abused are often aroused by their behaviour. However, the 'acting out' behaviours described above may occur in other circumstances. Many teenagers have low self-esteem, and acting out behaviour alone or early sexual activity are insufficient grounds for enquiry at the outset. Routine questions about abuse are not helpful.[8] There is a danger that, once denied, the subject cannot be broached again when the teenager feels more comfortable or confident with the healthcare worker. Children who have run away from home often give vague responses to questions about their reasons, such as 'I was fed up'. A study from a safe house provided by the Children's Society found that one in five children had suffered sexual abuse before running away.[9] Similarly, given time to establish that their concerns will be heard in a calm and non-judgemental way, teenagers can often divulge their hidden problems.

Health professionals can give signals that they are willing to hear about abusive situations. Enquire about the age of the partner, especially when the very young attend for contraception; 12- and 13-year-olds are fortunately not often clients at clinics, and even less often at general practice surgeries. However, it is not uncommon to discover that sexual activity is occurring in this age group with a much older male, and issues of child protection then have to be discussed. Disparity of age (e.g. the 15-year-old girl with a 30-year-old man) will raise concern about power imbalance and abuse with 14- and 15-year-olds, too.

A 13-year-old girl told her mother that she had been having sex with a 17-year-old boy for three weeks. The mother and daughter attended the clinic together with a request for the girl to go on the pill as she had just started her period. The mother's concern was that her daughter did not get pregnant. The girl was sulky and defiant. She did not see why she should stop having sex and was definite that, as the boy would not use condoms, she must

continued

go on the pill. She denied that any coercion or pressure had been used to make her have sex. A difficult discussion with both the mother and the daughter, separately and together, about the legal position and the consequences did not appear to have any effect, except that the mother said she would have a word with the boy's mother. Neither wanted the intervention of Social Services or the police. The doctor felt that her first duty at this stage concerned the health of the girl and, after checking for contra-indications, she started the girl on the pill. Permission to contact the family's GP or the health visitor was sought but not given. The doctor arranged to see them again in two weeks after they had had a chance to think about what had been said, fearing that a more active approach would put them off attending the clinic in the future.

Health professionals may be alerted to the existence of abuse by certain problems presented by adolescents, such as the following psychosocial complaints:

- truancy
- anorexia
- disturbed, disruptive or aggressive behaviour
- self-harm
- obsessive behaviour (e.g. repeated washing)
- emotionally withdrawn behaviour
- drug use
- loss of concentration
- loss of bowel or bladder control.

Physical complaints may include the following:

- anal pain or bleeding
- vaginal pain, soreness or discharge
- perineal soreness
- sexually transmitted infections

- signs of trauma
- almost any psychosomatic complaint[10] (abdominal pain, joint pains, headaches, itching, etc.).

Adolescents may ask openly for help at a time of crisis or change. A daughter may reveal that she has been abused when a younger sister is about to supplant her in the special relationship that she has, partly endured and partly enjoyed. A girl may find that a developing relationship outside the closely knit family threatens to disrupt the arrangements within the family or expose another sibling to risk. Increasing maturity or living away from home for the first time may evoke the realisation that what has been happening is not a normal experience for others. Publicity in the media, the advertising of telephone helplines or teaching in schools and youth organisations may increase confidence to the point where a disclosure can be made. The need to cope with contraception (when no method is ever right) or with an intimate examination (when the time is never right) can provide the stimulus for broaching the subject. A new relationship or increasing self-confidence may open the door to revelations about previous experiences or risks at home.

What to do with the information

Probably the most important reaction for any recipient of information about abuse is to accept it and hear the person out. Stopping the flow of information, once the dam has been breached, sends a signal that the message cannot be tolerated. Similarly, expressions of horror or distress may make the adolescent pull back and feel that these matters are too terrible to discuss. An attitude of apparent calm acceptance by the healthcare worker helps victims of abuse to begin to realise that they too can bear the anger and distress.

It is important to recognise the powerlessness that is felt by people who have been abused. If the healthcare worker promptly takes over and organises a referral or starts telling that person what to do, the feelings of powerlessness are only reinforced. Allow the complainant to make their own decision in their own time as far as possible. A common finding is that the teenager does not want to do anything else once their situation has been told. It is almost as if the telling itself is the required action.

However, if anyone is currently at risk, time is of the essence, and counselling about the necessity of involving Social Services is mandatory. The healthcare worker should refer to the local guidelines about procedures. If the adolescent is in immediate danger, protective action must be taken and the police involved if necessary. If there is a case for investigation, referral to Social Services is made, if necessary via the emergency duty team. It is important to take care not to prejudice care or criminal proceedings, but to consider carefully the needs of the individual.

You may be asked to keep what you have been told completely confidential. You should always qualify any assurance you give about confidentiality with a caveat about the need to break confidentiality if the adolescent or other person is at serious risk of harm. Any plans that are made depend on an assessment of the adolescent's situation and that of their family. Immediate action can be taken, such as issuing a 'Place of Safety Order', and then a longer term plan can be made after a more comprehensive social and medical assessment. Keep good contemporaneous records, as they may be required many years in the future, and may also be needed for legal proceedings.

You may not have any direct information about abuse, but only suspicions. The imbalance of power between victim and abuser makes it imperative that other adults use their influence to support the adolescent. Observation and recording of visible injuries, writing down the stated age of the partner, and any reported evidence of abuse of power may all be helpful later if more concrete evidence is obtained. It also helps to alert others who may see the teenager on other occasions.

Rape and sexual assault

What it is (and isn't)

Violent sexual abuse of children and rape of adults have much in common. In both cases the perpetrator is in a position of power relative to the victim. Just as the child or adolescent is abused by the parent, older sibling or other adult, so the female (or male) who is sexually assaulted is subjugated by inequality of strength or fear of injury or death.

The general law on sexual intercourse (Sexual Offences Act 1956) states that there are two offences concerning a man who has sexual intercourse with a girl. These offences are committed *even if the girl consents*.

- It is an absolute offence for a man to have sexual intercourse with a girl under the age of 13 years. No defence of mistaking the age of the girl is allowed in this case.
- A man who has intercourse with a girl over 13 years but less than 16 years of age may be able to claim in his defence (and have to prove it on the balance of probabilities) that he believed her to be 16-years-old or over. This defence applies only if he is under 24-years-old and has not previously been charged with a similar offence.

The male is still committing an offence even if both are under 16-years-old or if he is younger than the girl. In practice, prosecutions are rare in the absence of evidence of exploitation or coercion. The Crown Prosecution Service is expected to act in the public interest, not just in the interests of an individual. Crown prosecutors are expected to consider the interests of a young person when deciding whether it is in the public interest to prosecute. The stigma of a conviction can cause serious harm to a boy or young man. However, the seriousness of the offence or the offender's past behaviour may make prosecution necessary, and prosecution should not be avoided just because of the offender's age.

Women and children are still considered by many to be the possessions of men, who regard themselves as able to do what they wish with them. In England, until recently the law still followed the guidelines from 1736 that 'the husband cannot be guilty of rape committed by himself upon his lawful wife, for by their mutual consent and contract the wife has given herself up in kind to her husband, which she cannot retract'. The Criminal Justice and Public Order Act 1994 amended the definition of rape by:

- making it clear that a husband can be guilty of the rape of his wife if she does not consent to sexual intercourse
- extending the law of rape to cover anal intercourse with a woman
- extending the law of rape to cover anal intercourse with a man.

Sexual intercourse must occur without consent for it to be classed as rape. Force, fear or fraud does not need to be exercised, and consent is given the meaning that she (or he) wishes to have sexual intercourse. It does not imply submission, and she (or he) must understand the 'nature of the act'. Rape is now defined by the Sexual Offences Act of 1956, amended as described above, as follows.

1 It is an offence for a man to rape a woman or another man.
2 A man commits rape if:

- he has sexual intercourse (whether vaginal or anal) with a person who at the time of intercourse does not consent to it and
- at the time he knows that the person does not consent to the intercourse or he is reckless as to whether the person consents to it.

The law defines sexual intercourse as demanding penetration by the man's penis, and it need not include ejaculation. Other forms of penetration are classed as sexual assault.

The old rule that a boy under 14 years of age was presumed incapable of intercourse was abolished by the Criminal Justice Act 1993, and a boy of any age may now be found guilty of any of the offences involving sexual assault or rape.

There are many myths about rape. It is widely believed that women have enjoyable fantasies about rape, and many men have difficulty in accepting that women who do have such fantasies do not wish to carry them out. Fantasies about being chased or forced may come from deep within the subconscious and may be enjoyable, exciting or erotic. The reality is very different. Rape is not enjoyable – it is degrading, frightening and violent.

Jokes about rape mask the reality of what it involves. It is a crime of violence and frequently involves beating, physical restraint, the use of weapons, urinating or defecating on to the victim or other forms of degradation. Victims are frequently afraid that they will be killed, and may continue to fear that this will happen after the event if they divulge what has happened. The fear and degradation parallel the feelings experienced during childhood sexual abuse.

Another widely held myth is that rape is carried out by maniacs who roam the streets. This is similar to the belief that abusers of children are mentally abnormal individuals who are easily recognisable as such. In most cases of both rape and sexual abuse, the abuser is known to the victim. It is also commonly believed that only certain types of women are raped, and that the rapist is in the grip of an uncontrollable sexual urge. However, it can be shown that most rapes are planned and the assault will be postponed if the circumstances are unfavourable to the perpetrator. Statistics from the London Rape Crisis Centre[11] showed that the assailant was known to the woman in over 50% of reported rapes, and that 60% of women were raped inside a building, and 30% in their own homes.

Reactions of the victim to rape and sexual violence

The reactions of the victim to sexual violation are similar regardless of the age at which such violation occurs. Burgess and Halstrom identified what they described as the 'rape trauma syndrome'. There is an initial acute phase in which physical symptoms predominate. These consist of the injuries sustained in the assault and the physical manifestations of anxiety. They include muscle tension, sleep disturbance, and gastrointestinal irritability with pain, anorexia and nausea. Genito-urinary symptoms of vaginal discharge, cystitis and pelvic pain or rectal pain or bleeding may occur.

In the second phase the victim reorganises their life. They may move away to a different area or avoid anyone except a few trusted close friends and family. Fear of anywhere reminiscent of the location where the assault took place may restrict their activities.

> A 16-year-old girl had just started work in a local town, and was travelling there and back each day by bus. She was dragged into a churchyard and raped whilst walking from work to the bus station one winter evening. She was able to resume her work and appeared outwardly calm, but was totally unable to walk to the bus station by herself. If she tried to do so she broke down in a panic attack.

Sexual fears emerge and sexual relationships are often compromised. An outward appearance of being well adjusted may belie the underlying denial and distress.

During the third phase the victim becomes depressed and needs to talk about the events. Anxieties also reappear at this stage. This phase may be triggered by a court appearance, particularly if the victim is made to feel like the person who is on trial. If the man is not convicted or receives a trivial sentence, she may feel guilt or responsibility together with a fear of a recurrence. Those women who were unable to resist (the 'frozen rabbit' response) at the time of the attack seem most likely to be seriously troubled about their role in the assault.

The pattern of symptoms that occur in childhood sexual abuse almost exactly mirrors the symptoms described above. Hobbs and Wynne[12] have described sleep disturbance, abdominal pain, changes in appetite and anxiety symptoms (the first phase). Edwards and Donaldson[5] include in their description of incest-survivor symptoms identical problems to those mentioned earlier, including sexual relationship problems, depression, lack of self-esteem, communication difficulties, self-destructive behaviour, feelings of shame or guilt, and anger and hostility.

Those who have been affected by childhood sexual abuse and who exhibit the reactions outlined above are more at risk of forced sexual activity as adults as part of the general exploitation to which they have become accustomed. They do not know how to protest against it, nor do they understand that they should do so. Their low self-esteem and guilt about having been despoiled and violated prevent them from protesting or asserting themselves in the future.

How to help the victims

One of the most important factors in recovering from sexual assault is to be able to talk about what happened and how it feels. Victims feel both helpless and worthless. They are unable to ask for help because of a lack of self-esteem (why should anyone listen to me?) or they deny that it has actually happened, as in any disaster (if I don't think about it I will wake up from this nightmare and find that it has not happened). They may become so angry that listeners cannot tolerate the emotions that are being expressed, unless they have been trained to do so.

People who have been sexually assaulted want to wash immediately afterwards. They need to know that they should not wash until samples have been obtained to provide evidence. They should take a change of clothes to the examination, as the clothes they were wearing will be retained. They also need to be screened for sexually transmitted infections and to have protection with emergency contraception. Follow-up arrangements should be made. Some areas of the country have rape examination suites where a less clinical atmosphere helps to make people feel more at ease, and there may be showers available for use after the examination. Efforts have been made to provide women police officers with special training, and to provide female police surgeons.

Referral to a rape crisis centre can be very helpful. Most of them are run by women for women, and they provide an environment in which victims can control the level of contact that is made. They can take what they need, ranging from telephone contact to full non-judgemental support in a group or from an individual. Rape crisis centres can arrange referrals to lawyers or specialised housing agencies. They will also give support and accompany victims to police stations, courts and clinics as necessary.

Those who become very distressed may need referral for individual help from psychologists, psychiatric services or sexual therapy clinics. Males who have been sexually assaulted often need specialised help, especially as rape crisis centres are orientated to provide help for women only.

A young woman had moved back to her parental home after being raped in her student lodgings by an ex-boyfriend. Her mother or father accompanied her whenever she left the house, at first with her willing consent, but later she found their protectiveness suffocating. They found a young man who was the son of close friends of theirs who they felt would be a suitable substitute. However, on their first date he tried to force her into having sex with him, and she subsequently made a suicide attempt, believing that all men would behave like this in future.

Victims should not have to find that their feelings of helplessness are being compounded by being 'taken over' by support services. They need to be encouraged in their autonomy to ask for help when it is needed and to work through their feelings at their own pace. Often those on the sidelines try to make those who have been affected deny that they are still suffering ('Surely you should be over it by now?') in order to minimise their own distress at what has happened. Other individuals may become over-protective and make the victim feel even less in control of her or his life (and paradoxically more likely to suffer a recurrence).

> A man consulted his doctor complaining that he had completely gone off sexual activity with his wife. It emerged that his brother had recently been convicted of raping a young woman at work. He knew this woman, had found her attractive, and could not imagine how his own brother could behave like that with someone who 'was not like that'. His feelings of horror at the effects of uncontrolled sexual activity had affected his own relationship.

Prevention

Neighbourhood schemes or projects to improve parenting skills can help young or inexperienced parents to learn how to avoid situations in which abuse may occur. Specific help for people who have been victims can help to prevent a cycle of abuse.

Children at school can learn about the boundaries of permitted touching. They need to know that they have a right to control access to their bodies, and that certain ways of being touched are unacceptable. They have to learn to trust their own feelings about what is acceptable. They need to be able to say 'no' and know how to tell another adult if they have been touched in an unacceptable way. Moreover, they must be heard, not dismissed, if they do tell someone.

Increased awareness that the home is the area of greatest risk for sexual assault, and that almost all abusers are not overtly mentally ill, can help potential victims to recognise the dangers more clearly. Training in self-esteem and assertiveness can help adolescents to state what is acceptable for them. Having a goal to work towards and a sense of their own identity makes young people less obvious targets for abuse or exploitation. Learning self-defence techniques not only provides a useful skill, but often also helps to develop self-esteem and a sense of control over previously feared situations.

Health professionals have an important role to play. They can be aware of the problems that present as signs of abuse or assault, they can refer parents for help with their parenting skills, and they also need to acknowledge that children have rights and responsibilities which gradually increase as they grow older. Assuming that a parent can give permission for a child to be examined perpetuates the loss of autonomy. The older the child, the more important it is that he or she is involved in the decision making. Agreement should be obtained from both the parent and the child, unless the urgency of the condition prevents this. Give an explanation to the child that is appropriate to their age when an examination involves touching a part of the body that is not usually touched by others. Explain the reasons why it is acceptable under these particular circumstances (e.g. that the touching is done for medical reasons and in the presence of a parent or nurse).

Physical examination of healthy young adolescents for contraception should be restricted to the minimum necessary from the history, and usually only includes a blood pressure reading, not a pelvic examination. Taking swabs or other invasive procedures should always be preceded by the patient's full informed consent.

Everyone has a responsibility to respect the autonomy of others. No human being should be used violently by another or for selfish sexual gratification. Sexual abuse or exploitation should be unacceptable. However, sexual assault can arouse strong emotions such as disgust, excitement or a desire for retribution. Apostolic fervour – religious or social (including excessive feminism) – can manifest itself as a desire to convert everyone to the cause of diagnosing abuse, to the detriment of individuals. In contrast, attitudes that are too authoritarian or cynical may fail a complainant. Over-identification with an abuser or a victim can prevent logical thought. Healthcare workers and others in contact with adolescents need to examine their own attitudes and skills in order to work with them as effectively as possible.

The field of abuse and sexual assault is full of challenges that present major ethical dilemmas for us all.

References

1 Kempe RS and Kempe CH (1978) *Child Abuse*. Fontana/Open Books, London.

2 Jones DPH and McQuiston MG (1988) *Interviewing the Sexually Abused Child*. Royal College of Psychiatrists, London.

3 Skruse D, Bentovim A, Hodges J *et al.* (1988) Risk factors for development of sexually abusive behaviour in sexually victimised adolescent boys: cross-sectional study. *BMJ.* **317**: 175–9.

4 Tsai M, Feldman-Summers S and Edgar M (1979) Childhood molestation: variables related to differential impacts on psychosocial functioning in adult women. *J Abnorm Psychol.* **88**: 407–17.

5 Edwards PW and Donaldson MA (1989) Assessment of symptoms in adult survivors of incest. *Child Abuse Neglect.* **13**: 101–10.

6 Fiscella K, Kitzman HJ, Cole RE, Sidora KJ and Olds D (1998) Does child abuse predict adolescent pregnancy? *Pediatrics.* **101**: 620–24.

7 Edgardh K, Krogh G and Ormstad K (1999) Adolescent girls investigated for sexual abuse: history, physical findings. *Forens Sci Int.* **104**: 1–15 (review).

8 Wakley G (1991) *Sexual Abuse and the Primary Care Doctor*. Chapman & Hall, London.

9 The Children's Society (1989) *Young Runaways: findings from Britain's first safe house*. The Children's Society, London.

10 Jehu D (1988) *Beyond Sexual Abuse*. John Wiley & Sons, Chichester.

11 The London Rape Crisis Centre (1984) *Sexual Violence*. The Women's Press, London.

12 Hobbs CJ and Wynne JM (1987) Management of sexual abuse. *Arch Dis Child*. **62**: 1182–7.

► CHAPTER 14

Influence on teenagers of peers, the media and the press

By the time young people reach adolescence they have learned sexual attitudes, values and behaviours and picked up gender stereotypes. Girls tend to believe that they should fit in with what men want in the way of a feminine image, believing that 'romance' and 'being in love' are important. Boys adopt a competitive masculine style and believe that risk-taking is part of 'being a man'. They may regard being ready and willing for sex as being part of that male persona.[1]

Women's experience of sexuality does not fit into either of the two extremes – of a whore with sexual feelings or a pure maiden with no sexual feelings at all. Bombarded as they are with images, clichés and media distortions, it is hardly surprising that young people are confused. Their attempts to create their own sexual identity leave them feeling exposed and vulnerable to criticism.

Traditional roles for women are similarly confused, particularly by the media's representations of how they should behave. Women see their bodies, particularly young attractive bodies, exploited as a commodity to sell almost everything. Women's bodies are presented as objects that must conform to criteria of being thin, spotless and dressed in designer clothing. Teenagers feel that they cannot achieve this ideal, as many of them are naturally plump, with acne and on a low income so unable to purchase fashionable clothes. There is no place here either for the teenager in a wheelchair or with a hearing aid. Their identity as women is not confirmed, just as the picture of the man as the breadwinner can no longer be sustained.

Peers

Peer education is heralded as a key influence and positive force in many current schemes to reduce teenage pregnancy rates, and has already been described in earlier chapters.

The extent of regretted first intercourse highlights the significant negative pressures that many youngsters are under from their peers to embark on sexual activity.[2,3] In total, 30 (7%) of 458 women reported being forced to have intercourse on the first occasion, with rates of reported coercion increasing with younger age at first intercourse.[2]

Television

Television is thought to help young people to define cultural norms, and it influences their perceptions of the real world and acceptable social behaviour.[4] Television, radio, newspapers and magazines are all popular media for delivering preventive health messages, and are often regarded as appropriate ways to engage young people.

The influence of the media and of advertising has been blamed as one of the contributory factors that encourage teenagers to become sexually active at an earlier age.[5]

A national omnibus survey of American parents and teenagers conducted in 1999[6] explored parents' views about 'who or what influences your teen child or children most, besides their boyfriend or girlfriend, when it comes to decisions about sex'. It was found that 11% thought that 'television, movies and musicians' exerted the most influence on their teenage offspring, compared to 55% who thought that parents or guardians had most influence; 14% believed that peers were most influential and 13% considered religion to carry most weight. When young people themselves were asked the same question, 8% thought that 'television, movies and musicians' had most influence on their decisions about sex, as opposed to parents or guardians (38%), peers (25%) and religion (14%). The majority of the parents and teenagers considered that teachers had little influence on teenagers' decision making about sex, with 0.3% of parents and 2% of teenagers believing that teachers were the most important figures in young people's lives with regard to influencing their decisions about sexual behaviour.

The power of the media to influence teenagers' behaviour has been demonstrated by health promotion campaigns such as that shown in the box below.[4,7] Both the intensity of the messages and the duration over which they are delivered appear to be important. The authors of one particular study believed that the mass media was a particularly appropriate vehicle for relaying health promotion messages, which were regarded as more credible when relayed via the mass media as opposed to school programmes, and because high-risk youngsters were extensively exposed to and interested in the media. A British Audience Research Bureau report showed that 4 to 15-year-olds watched an average of 19 hours of television per week, and 16- to 24-year-olds watched 20 hours of television per week.

Smoking prevention messages presented via the mass media can have large and durable effects on high-risk adolescents. The 'mass media' used was an average of 540 television and 350 radio broadcasts per year for four years, with health promotion relayed in media programmes that were popular with targeted groups. The school-based intervention consisted of three or four lessons per year delivered by school teachers over the same period. A combination of mass media and school interventions was more effective than school-based interventions alone. The lower smoking rates among high-risk youngsters persisted when they were measured two years later.[7]

Radio

The evaluation of a week-long local radio campaign publicising emergency contraception found that 7% of the 200 people who were questioned afterwards had noted the campaign. Of those 7%, half were subsequently fully informed of both hormonal and intrauterine methods of emergency contraception and the time within which they were effective. Although the small number who had learned about emergency contraception through the campaign was disappointing, the extent of their knowledge heartened the authors of the study.[8]

Teen idols

Britney Spears is an American pop star who, at the age of 18 years, is a teenage idol. She publicly declared that she was committed to celibacy until her wedding night. She is thought to have made this high-profile declaration in order to provide encouragement to girls and young women who find themselves under pressure from boyfriends to give in to sexual demands. In America, self-declared teenage celibates are known as 'pledge-keepers'.[9]

The Internet

The Internet is generally regarded as a useful resource that has the potential to supply information about health to aid understanding and empower the individual in any medical consultation. This bodes well for the young person who is seeking information about sexuality or contraception – so long as the information is accurate and reliable. However, sexual health promotion via the Internet may be more open to abuse than any other health topic. Sexual health sites may be accessed by children (for whom explicit material is unsuitable) or exploited by pornographers or extremists. The following Health

Education Authority principles are intended to safeguard the use of the Internet for sexual health promotion:[10]

- make sure that all communications are accompanied by a detailed brief explaining what public health outcomes and health impact are intended
- recognise the diversity of sexual attitudes and sexual lifestyles, and avoid being judgemental
- promote mutual self-respect, and the benefits to well-being that are derived from caring and emotionally fulfilling relationships
- messages should be accurate, clear and honest in cases where there is uncertainty about the evidence
- the target audience should be carefully defined
- the language should be justified by its purpose and intended outcome
- all materials should be pretested and modified in response to research findings before being released on to the Internet.

Magazines

Magazines were judged to be an important source of information in a study that sought to understand the factors which influence young people in their sexual behaviour and their attitudes towards pregnancy.[11] Problem pages were regarded as being particularly useful.

Places where teenagers can go for advice – the teenager's perspective

The following commentary by Steph reports the views of her contemporaries

Teenagers need a confidential and non-embarrassing way to obtain information about different aspects of sex.

continued

One such method is the use of teenage magazines. Magazines explain different subjects that a teenager may be thinking about, and sex and teenage pregnancy are just two of them. They have articles and problem pages where they give expert advice. This resource is very appealing because it is not embarrassing to buy, as it is full of many different articles, and no one has to know why you have bought it. Magazines provide an easy and effective way to find things out, and they deal with teenage issues very well. They are reasonably cheap, ranging from about 90p to £2.00 an issue.

It is mainly girls who read the information, but some girls say that boys in their class at school have taken their magazines when they were not looking and read them.

The one problem with magazines is that if you were in trouble and were already pregnant, then they probably would not tell you what you needed to know. After all, a magazine cannot specialize in every subject every week. They are normally published monthly and are not a quick source of information.

Commercial advertisements

Bellis and Ashton have suggested that one effective way to influence cultural attitudes that has not been tried so far is via commercial advertisements in the media.[12] They argue that promoting condoms or particular condom brands should increase their acceptability to young people, by altering the image of condoms and extending the market. The two public health leaders are pleading for a revision to restrictive legislation on commercial advertising, which is based on anxieties about the possibility that advertising products such as condoms could promote promiscuity.

References

1   Aggleton P, Oliver C and Rivers K (1998) *Reducing the Rate of Teenage Conceptions – the Implications of Research into Young People, Sex, Sexuality and Relationships.* Health Education Authority, London.

2   Dickson N, Paul C, Herbison P *et al.* (1998) First sexual intercourse: age, coercion, and later regrets reported by a birth cohort. *BMJ.* **316**: 29–33.

3   Wight D, Henderson M, Raab G *et al.* (2000) Extent of regretted sexual intercourse among young teenagers in Scotland: a cross-sectional survey. *BMJ.* **320**: 1243–4.

4   NHS Centre for Reviews and Dissemination (1999) *Preventing the Uptake of Smoking in Young People.* Effective Health Care Bulletin. Volume 5. Royal Society of Medicine, London.

5   Bury J (1984) *Teenage Pregnancy in Britain.* Birth Control Trust, London.

6   National Campaign to Prevent Teen Pregnancy (1999) *National Omnibus Survey.* National Campaign to Prevent Teen Pregnancy, Washington, DC.

7   Flynn B, Worden J, Secker-Walker R *et al.* (1997) Long-term responses of higher- and lower-risk youths to smoking prevention interventions. *Prevent Med.* **26**: 389–94.

8   Desmond N, Whitlow B and Hay P (1995) A publicity campaign for emergency contraception. *Br J Fam Plan.* **21**: 154.

9   Harlow J (2000) Pop princess sets her heart on celibacy. *The Sunday Times.* **14 May**: 26.

10 Health Education Authority (1998) *Sexual Health in Cyberspace. Overcoming the Obstacles to Promoting Sexual Health on the Internet.* Health Education Authority, London.

11 Health Education Authority (1999) *Reducing the Rate of Teenage Conceptions. Summary Bulletin. Young People's Experiences of Relationships, Sex and Early Parenthood: Qualitative Research.* Health Education Authority, London.

12 Bellis M and Ashton J (2000) Commercial advertisements are needed to create a condom culture. *BMJ.* **320**: 643.